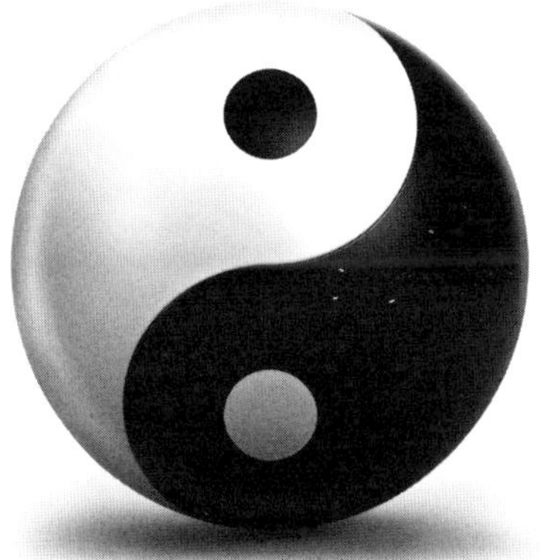

BY THE SAME AUTHOR

Arms, Armour & the Tactics of Warfare (Book of Samurai series, Book 2)
Book of Ninja: The First Complete Translation of the Bansenshukai
Fundamental Samurai Teachings (Book of Samurai series, Book 1)
How to Be a Modern Samurai: 10 Steps to Finding Your Power & Achieving Success
Iga and Koka Ninja Skills: The Secret Shinobi Scrolls of Chikamatsu Shigenori
In Search of the Ninja: The Historical Truth of Ninjutsu
Modern Ninja Warfare: Tactics and Methods for the Modern Warrior
Ninja Skills: The Authentic Ninja Training Manual
Old Japan: Secrets From the Shores of the Samurai
Samurai and Ninja: The Real Story Behind the Japanese Warrior Myth That Shatters the Bushido Mystique
Samurai War Stories
Secrets of the Ninja: The Shinobi Teachings of Hattori Hanzo
The Dark Side of Japan: Ancient Black Magic, Folklore, Ritual
The Illustrated Guide to Viking Martial Arts
The Lost Samurai School: Secrets of Mubyoshi Ryu
The Lost Warfare of India: An Illustrated Guide
The Secret Traditions of the Shinobi: Hattori Hanzo's Shinobi Hiden and Other Ninja Scrolls
The Ultimate Art of War: A Step-by-Step Illustrated Guide to the Teachings of Sun Tzu
True Path of the Ninja: The Definitive Translation of the Shoninki

THE ULTIMATE GUIDE TO
YIN YANG

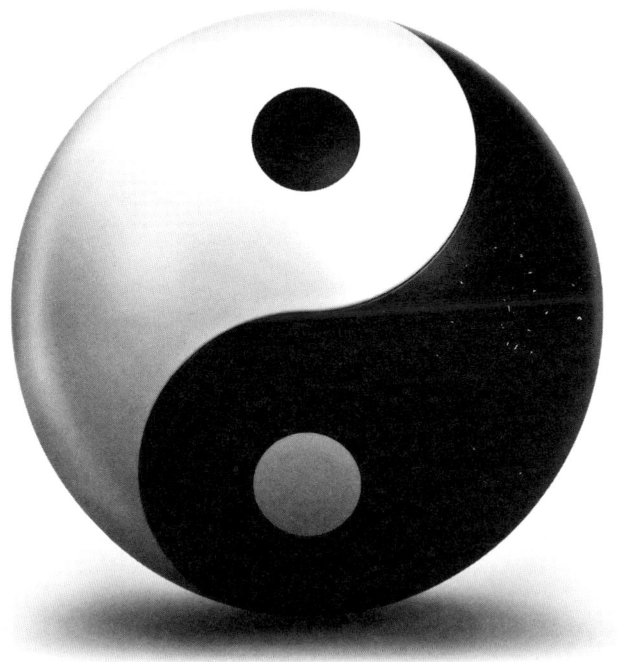

AN ILLUSTRATED EXPLORATION OF THE CHINESE CONCEPT OF OPPOSITES

ANTONY CUMMINS

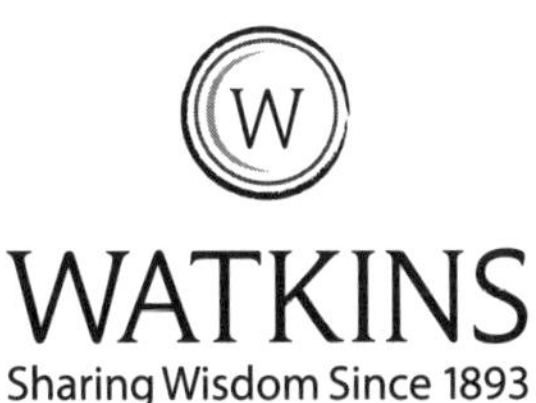
WATKINS
Sharing Wisdom Since 1893

THE ULTIMATE GUIDE TO YIN YANG

ANTONY CUMMINS

This edition first published in the UK and USA in 2021 by
Watkins, an imprint of Watkins Media Limited
Unit 11, Shepperton House
89–93 Shepperton Road
London N1 3DF

enquiries@watkinspublishing.com

Commissioning Editor: Fiona Robertson
Editor: James Hodgson
Head of Design: Glen Wilkins
Designer: Luise Roberts
Production Manager: Uzma Taj

Commissioned Artwork: Jay Kane

A CIP record for this book is available from the British Library.

ISBN: 978-1-78678-515-2 (Hardback)
ISBN: 978-1-78678-551-0 (eBook)

10 9 8 7 6 5 4 3 2 1

Printed in China

www.watkinspublishing.com

To Ben McCarty
for his support of my projects

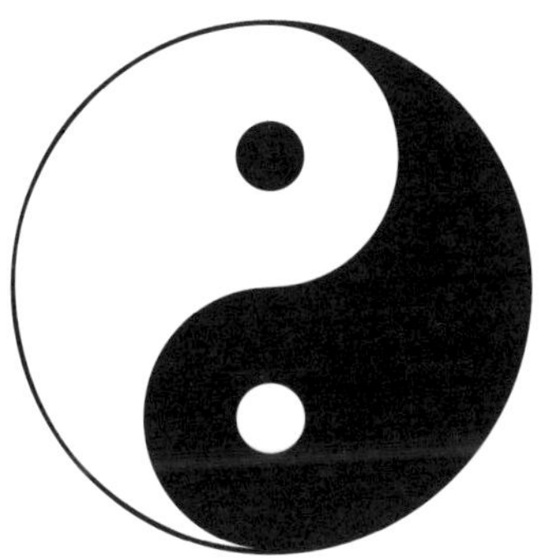

In spite of common assumptions about yinyang,
its main function is not about describing
the world or its origins, but rather in
enabling one to live well in it.

Robin Wang

ACKNOWLEDGEMENTS

I am indebted to Robin Wang, whose outstanding book *Yinyang: The Way of Heaven and Earth in Chinese Thought and Culture* was the wedge that broke yinyang open for me. For those people who want to delve deeper into the subject, I could not recommend his book strongly enough. I must also thank Élisabeth Rochat de la Vallée, whose book *Yin Yang in Classical Texts* is a great way to understand the evolution of the concept as it progressed through the ages. Thanks also to Monkey Press, who kindly sent me books to support my project. Thanks also to Les Conn for help with aspects of Chinese pronouncation and to Derek Yuen for his help with Chinese ideograms. Also to Ikenaga Yukiko for her help with Japanese ideograms and pronunciations. To Mieko Koizumi for her guidance and support in all such matters. Lastly, to James Hodgson, my editor, for his tireless work, and Fiona Robertson of Watkins Publishing for her stalwart support in all my ventures and for bringing this book to reality.

CONTENTS

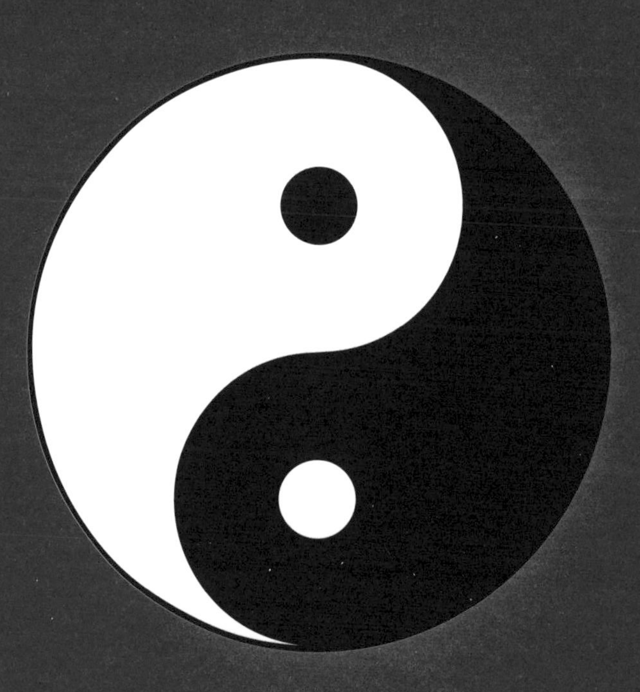

INTRODUCTION: A STORY OF OPPOSITES

LIVING WITH YINYANG

From the dawn of Chinese civilization yinyang has shaped nations and peoples and this eternal symbol of balance and harmony continues to have a powerful presence today. People all over the world live with its teachings in mind to achieve greater balance. However, following the correct path within the restrictions of human society is a constant struggle.

In a perfect world, each person would have abundant land, benefit from the fruits of the earth, rise with the sun and look up at the bright moon. Family and friends would gather round the warmth of a wood fire as the bounty of earth kept everyone safe within its bosom while the sky watched overhead. Sadly, this cannot always be so; while modern living has great benefits, it can be difficult to arrange your life according to ancient principles in today's world.

However, all people can enhance their lives by following the teachings of yinyang. By doing so, they can establish greater balance not only in their own world but also the world at large as they work together with other people to follow nature's flow. Attach yourself to the deeper secrets of the ancient sage masters of China and engage in a new way with an old tradition.

A NEW WAY OF HARMONY

Yin and yang: two words that have entered into the world consciousness and seeped their meaning into many aspects of life. There are few people who do not recognize yin and yang, yet most people only understand the concept as a vague idea of opposites. While many books have yinyang in their title, most just use it as a shorthand for balance within a given theme – the yinyang of painting, the yinyang of cooking, and so on. There are very few books dedicated to the study of yinyang itself, and they tend to be too academic and complex for the casual reader who comes to the subject with limited prior knowledge.

The aim of all my work is to bring complex ideas to a wider audience without losing the richness of the subject, and this book is no different. It opens up a gateway into the mysterious world of yinyang and gives you two paths to follow. The first leads you to a solid historical understanding of the origins and evolution of yinyang; the second is a way to use these ancient teachings in your own life, to follow the sage masters of old and benefit from the bounty of the eternal Dao.

From the basic concepts and historical development of yinyang through to its uses and skills, the book will outline all you need to know about harmonizing with the Way and help you position yourself in life so that you can benefit from the abundance of the universe. This is not a path of laziness; it is one that shows you how to ride the waves of existence and land on the shores of contentment.

At the end of each chapter you will find a "Working with yinyang" box, which comprises a short meditation on the key learnings of that chapter. Often it will encourage you to look at the landscape around you, the sky overhead or the development of your own understanding and reflect on the immense power and beauty of yinyang in action.

A BASIS FOR OTHER SUBJECTS

Some people study Traditional Chinese Medicine or herb lore, *qi gong* or martial arts; others are drawn to samurai battle strategy, *shiatsu*, Japanese massage, omens and portents, acupuncture, acupressure, lucky and unlucky directions, and so on. These subjects all have one thing in common: they require an understanding of yinyang.

Therefore, if you have an interest in east Asian thought and culture in general or one of these practices in particular you will benefit from reading this book, even if you did not set out to learn about yinyang in the first place.

BEFORE YOU BEGIN

When approaching any ancient Chinese subject, there are certain difficulties that can trip you up if you are not aware of them. These include the complex problem of translating ideas from one language, culture and era to another. It is easy to make incorrect assumptions based on our western understanding of concepts such as spirit, soul and heaven. Therefore, before we start we will look at some of the most common stumbling blocks.

CHINESE WORDS

The intricacies of yinyang are difficult enough to grasp on their own without having to deal with a foreign language. For this reason, I have tried to avoid bombarding you with Chinese terms. However, if we stray too far from the original Chinese terminology there is a deep danger of misinterpreting important concepts and giving birth to various inaccuracies. Therefore, any Chinese terms used in this book will be accompanied by their English translation and in many cases the original Chinese ideogram.

To compound the problem, Chinese can be transliterated in two ways: using either the Wade-Giles system or the Pinyin system. The Wade-Giles version came first, but then in the twentieth century the Chinese turned to Pinyin as the official system for saying and spelling Chinese words across the world. This has meant that well-established names and concepts have had to be relearned. For example, the Tao and Taoism in Wade-Giles became the Dao and Daoism in Pinyin; the legendary military tactician Sun Tzu became Sunzi; the universal life force *chi* became *qi*; and the famous manual the Tao Te Ching became the Dao De Jing. In this book I will use a mixture of the two systems, because certain words are more popular in one version than the other. For example, I will use the Dao instead of the Tao, but *chi* instead of *qi*. Where appropriate, I will also give Japanese terms alongside their Chinese counterparts.

However, do not get too bogged down in the language. First understand the meaning of the concepts and then later, if you like, you can gain a deeper appreciation by engaging with the original Chinese characters.

THE SOUL AND SPIRIT

The terms "soul" and "spirit" are used interchangeably throughout this book to refer to the essence of a human beyond the physical body. They are approximations of the Chinese concept of the multi-part soul (see opposite) and do not have their precise Christian connotations.

A key difference is that the ancient Chinese believed that the soul of a human was divided into five basic components, itemized in the table opposite.

THE FIVE PARTS OF THE SOUL – *WUSHEN* (五神)				
NAME	IDEOGRAM	ASPECT	PLANET	DESCRIPTION
Shen	神	Fire	Mars	The upper spirit connected to heaven
Hun	魂	Wood	Jupiter	The yang part of the soul which ascends after death
Po	魄	Metal	Venus	The yin part of the soul which descends after death
Yi	意	Earth	Saturn	The intellectual and conceptual
Zhi	志	Water	Mercury	The will and intention

A SHARED CONCEPT

More often than not, yinyang is placed in the realm of Daoism, the Chinese religious and philosophical tradition that focuses on the Dao, or Way, the unknowable origin of all things. Daoism evolved from native thought traditions into a highly complex religion, with priests, holy sites and sophisticated ceremonies. It can be divided roughly speaking into two main factions: the philosophical Daoists, who debate the meaning of the Way; and the religious Daoists, who have a much more structured approach to the Way, involving ritual magic and high ceremony.

However, many eastern concepts, including yinyang, are shared by the whole culture rather than being held exclusively by a certain religion or thought tradition. Buddhists talk about the Dao even though it is essentially a Daoist concept and various religions use the terms *dharma* and *karma*. Yinyang predated Daoism and featured in folk religions throughout the ancient East, not all of which developed into Daoism. The theory would have been well understood by Chinese-speaking peoples throughout the region and continues to underpin the culture to this day.

Therefore, if you are coming to this book from a purely Daoist perspective, you may be surprised by the different angles from which yinyang can be viewed.

A NOTE ON SOURCES

All the research for this book was done from secondary sources listed in the Bibliography, most of which I found in the John Rylands Library at the University of Manchester. The books cover a wide range of subjects relating to yinyang and many quote from primary sources and ancient texts. For the sake of simplicity and flow, I have not referenced all the information included in this book. However, please understand that this information comes from identifiable and reputable academic sources, all of which can be found in the Bibliography.

ENJOY THE BOOK

For those who are interested, this book contains information on religious history, pronunciation, ideograms and numerous other subjects, but above all it is there to be enjoyed. In my journeys through eastern thought, from Traditional Chinese Medicine to Daoist philosophy via the esoteric teachings of the samurai, I have encountered yinyang at every step. However, I have never been able to find a book that explains yinyang in a simple way – and that is why I wrote *The Ultimate Guide to Yin Yang*. I hope that it will give the novice a solid foundation on which to base further investigation. And for those of you who are more familiar with the subject, I hope it will fill some gaps.

The Dao created the one, the one created the two, the two created three, the three contains all things in creation, and all of creation rests on yin and yang and the mixing of *chi* energy. This happened in the past, it is happening now and it will continue in the future.

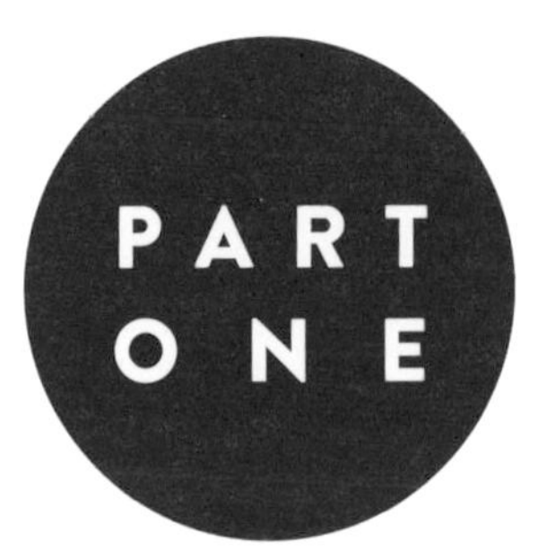

THE ESSENCE OF YINYANG

Before you race off into the ancient mountains of China, you need to understand the basic nature of yinyang – a subject that is often misunderstood. Part One takes a look at what yinyang actually is and how it works. This part of the book provides a foundation for the more complex understandings of yinyang that evolved over time, which are explored in Part Two.

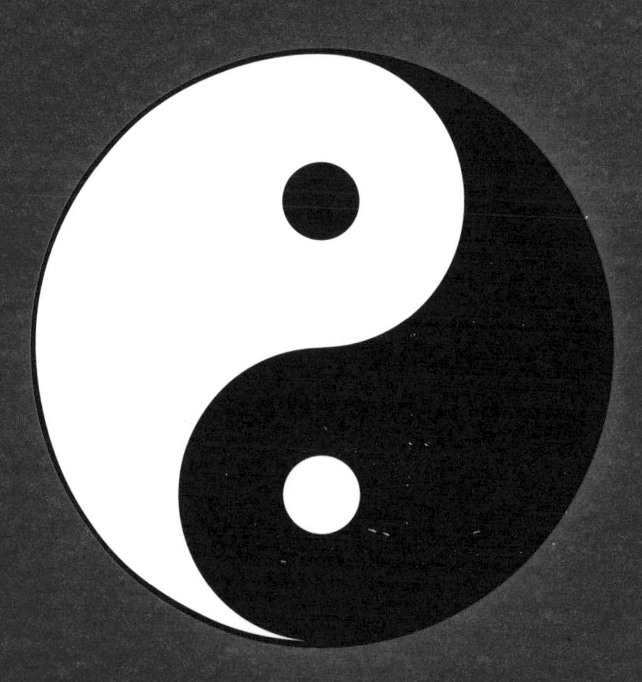

CHAPTER 1

UNDERSTANDING YINYANG

UNDERSTANDING YINYANG

Yinyang enables us to align ourselves with the universe so as to enhance our lives. By studying yinyang we can gain a better understanding of universal patterns, explain natural phenomena and, it is believed, predict and anticipate natural events. Yinyang is a manifestation of the Way (Dao) and a person who follows the Way rides on the universal laws of nature and "steals" the power of heaven.

THE GOAL OF YINYANG

The goal of yinyang can be broken down into the following areas:

- understanding the intellectual system of yinyang
- using *chi* as energy
- relying on the divine spirit within
- achieving longevity and purpose
- mastering the timing of heaven
- reaping the benefits of the earth
- entering into harmony with other humans

☯ **Those who follow the principles of yinyang will lead a life full of positive experiences in fruitful harmony with heaven, the world and other people.**

SAYING YINYANG

Everybody has heard of yinyang, but few people say it correctly. The right pronunciation is difficult for a western person to achieve and also differs depending on the period of Chinese history when the term is being used, and the area the speaker is from. In Cantonese, the pronunciation is "yam-yern", while in Mandarin it is "yin-yang" but with the "a" of the "yang" being close to an "o" and a very pronounced rise and fall of the two syllables. Be aware that the first part is "yin", not "ying" – this is a common mistake.

The sound is only the representation of an idea, not the idea itself.

WRITING YINYANG

People often write (and say) yin and yang separately. However, yinyang is a single concept consisting of two parts and as such it should be written as a single word. In this book, the two parts will only be written separately when we are referring to each part separately.

Yinyang is a single concept of two halves, not two separate ideas.

THE CHINESE CHARACTER FOR YIN

The traditional character for yin consists of three parts:

- hill
- today
- cloud

Together, these read as "the shadows of the clouds on the hill today".

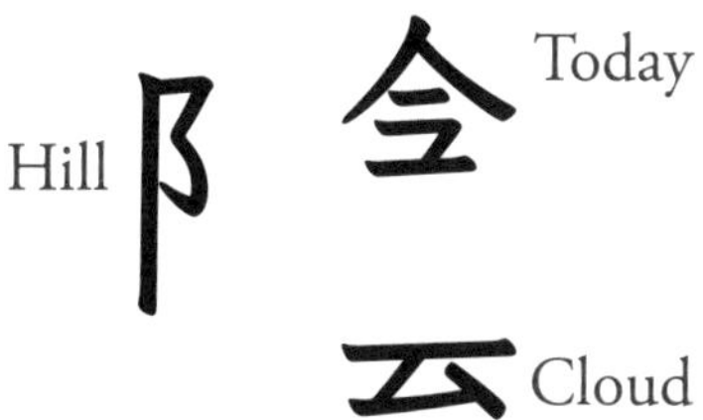

ABOVE: The traditional character for yin.

The cloud represents hidden, dark areas, such as crags, shadows and recesses. It is the shadow cast by the cloud that is significant rather than the cloud itself. This is the traditional image used for yin. However, the modern, simplified version of the character consists of just "hill" and "moon".

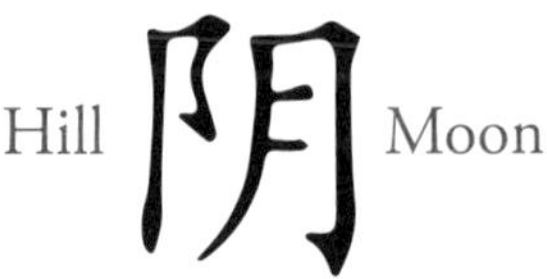

ABOVE: The modern ideogram for yin.

Yin is the rain, the cold and the shade. Perfect yin blasts and freezes.

THE CHINESE CHARACTER FOR YANG

The traditional character for yang consists of three parts:

- hill
- the sun coming over the horizon
- the light rays beaming off it

You can see the character for "sun" (日) with a line below it; this is the sun over the horizon with beams of light clearing the hills. Altogether this ideogram means "the rays of the sun that come over the horizon and touch the hills".

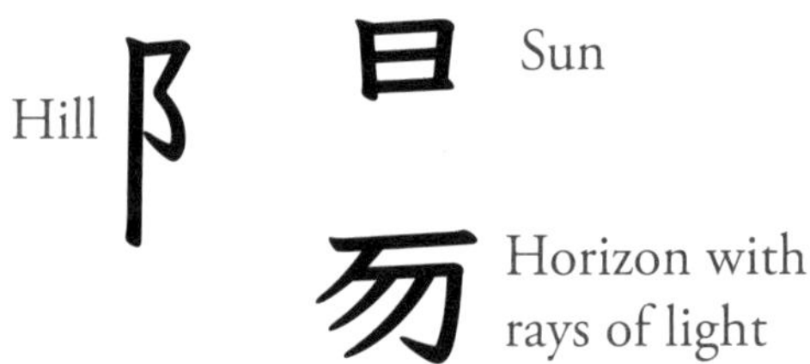

ABOVE: The traditional character for yang.

The bottom right part of the ideogram can also be interpreted as banners flying in the breeze on a bright, sunny day.

Like the traditional ideogram for yin, the ideogram for yang has been simplified for modern times. It now consists of "hill" and "sun".

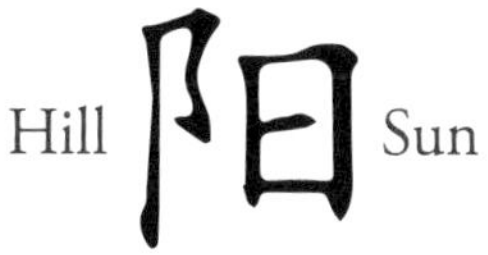

ABOVE: The modern ideogram for yang.

Yang is the dry, the heat and the bright. Perfect yang burns red hot.

THE SUN AND THE MOON

The sun and the moon are central to the concept of yinyang. The sun rises every day, ever steady, and never waxes or wanes. This is yang; it is full force. However, the moon's power varies in intensity according to its phases. This is yin; its power waxes and wanes.

Just as the sun and moon take turns to be in a position of power, so do yang and yin. However, yang power is always on full, while yin power comes and goes in subtle waves.

THE WORLD ABOVE AND BELOW

For the various peoples of ancient China, the universe was the earth below their feet and the sky above their heads. They saw themselves as having both a horizontal relationship with other people and also a vertical relationship with the heavens and whatever was beyond the stars. They called the sky *tian* (天) and they developed sophisticated systems to track the five known planets, the sun, the moon and smaller heavenly bodies such as comets. At the root of all these efforts was the simple idea that *chi* rose from the earth into the sky and also drifted down from heaven to the world below. This was yin and yang *chi* in action and humans were a part of that.

Tracking the movements of heavenly bodies gives a better understanding of the transfer of energy between heaven and earth.

ALL UNDER HEAVEN

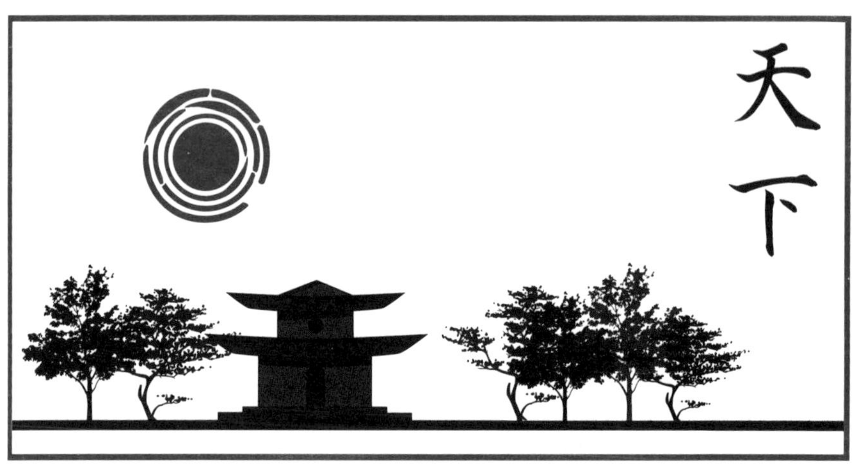

ABOVE: The ideogram for "all under heaven" consists of "sky" and "below".

The ancient Chinese used the term "all under heaven" to mean the world. The ideograms are "sky" and "below", as seen in the image above. This phrase is widely used and you may often read it in literature relating to Chinese culture. Earth was seen as serving heaven, and heaven was seen as directing worldly affairs. The sky was yang (associated with male) and the earth was yin (associated with female). Sometimes heaven was personified as a male emperor named Shang Di (上帝) who ruled the skies.

☯ **Everything on earth, including humans, serves the supernatural beings of heaven.**

WE ARE ALL EQUAL UNDER HEAVEN

We have seen that heaven has male associations and earth has female associations and that earth serves heaven. However, this does not mean that women serve men. Be careful not to make this mistake. All humans are equal to each other and equally subservient to the will of heaven in the eyes of the Dao.

THE CYCLE OF THE UNIVERSE

Galaxies spiral, planets orbit, the seasons come and go, day turns into night and night into day, flowers grow and die to grow again – all of the universe is cyclical. Sometimes yang will be predominant; at other times yin will be in control. The same land may be stricken by a raging fire or drought (yang) in summer and covered by snow or floodwater (yin) in winter. Yang is associated with life and yin with death. Neither one wins outright, nor do they fight; they simply pass control to each other in an endless cycle.

☯ **There will always be times when the world is either more yang or more yin, but it will return again either to equilibrium or to the opposite element.**

THE YINYANG MATRIX

The universe is made up of relationships between yin and yang *chi*. Known as the yinyang matrix, this network of energy channels holds existence in equilibrium. The ancient Chinese saw all of creation, from the positions of the stars and planets to the positioning of objects around the house, as dependent on the movements between yin and yang.

☯ **Yin and yang *chi* is constantly mutating and combining in countless ways to create existence.**

THE CHINESE UNDERSTANDING OF THE WORLD

Yinyang does not only govern the natural world but also infuses all of society, influencing areas such as systems of government, the design of cities and houses, human relationships and positions within the family. If all matters are in correct proportion and alignment, heaven's energy will flow correctly and human prosperity will increase. Conversely, if matters are in disarray, humans will suffer.

☯ The cosmos is always in motion but it is never in chaos. Only humans create chaos.

THE CONNECTION BETWEEN HEAVEN AND EARTH

The sun's rays cause both light and shadow to fall on the earth. Yin and yang are present in the sky in the form of the moon and the sun respectively. Yin and yang were the first movements in the universe and they continue to move from one state to the other and will do for all time.

☯ Yinyang was there at the beginning and it will be there at the end.

THE "TEN THOUSAND THINGS" CONNECT

The Chinese use the term "ten thousand things" (萬物) to refer to everything that is in creation, whether natural or made by humans. Yinyang is like a net that connects all things and holds them in place. Just like binary code, it consists of two components that can be combined in endless permutations. It is the fabric of reality, responsible for all things in creation.

☯ There is nothing in existence that is not some subtle blend of yin and yang, which create endless variations.

THE STARTING POINT FOR BOTH LIFE AND DEATH

Yinyang provides the initial spark for all things that are created. The movement between yin and yang causes *chi* to be held inside of something that until then had not existed.

To understand this, think of your hands when cold. There is only cold, but when you rub them together warmth is created. This "warmth" comes from the movement of yinyang.

However, all living beings must die. Yang is life and yin is death; yang moves into prominence at the start of life, but then life wanes and yin starts to take over. This eventually leads to death, destruction and dissipation, at which point the being's yang *chi* returns to the sky and its yin *chi* returns to the earth.

☯ Things emerge into the world with the power of yang and leave existence with the power of yin. Creation is a never-ending process.

YIN MAKES MATTER, YANG GIVES US NATURE

On a fundamental level, all yin energy makes matter and constructs the universe, bringing things to life. While yin creates something, yang is the nature inside of it, the identity and make-up of the structure. Yin is solid and dense; yang is light and radiates outward.

☯ The forces of yin and yang move together to create all things, but it is yin that forms their structure and yang that gives them their nature.

YINYANG IS THE WORSHIP OF REAL-WORLD PHENOMENA

In most religions there is a god to worship, or even a whole pantheon of deities arranged in a complex hierarchy. However, yinyang is the worship of natural phenomena, such as the wind, rain, sky, earth and stars. While China does have creation myths, the main Daoist version simply talks about yin and yang springing from the Great Ultimate. The Chinese do, of course, attach great spiritual significance to all these natural elements, but they do not personify them to the level other religious ways do.

☯ The Dao or the One is a form of consciousness; it does not have a backstory.

VERTICAL, HORIZONTAL AND CIRCULAR RELATIONSHIPS

In the Dao all things are interconnected. The three main forms of relationship are vertical, horizontal and circular.

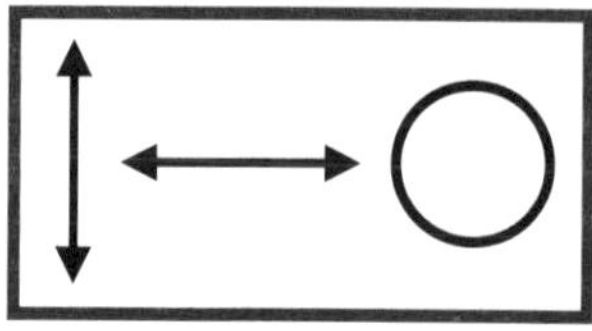

ABOVE:
The three forms of relationship: vertical, horizontal and circular.

- Vertical relationships are the ones humans have with heaven and earth.
- Horizontal relationships are between all things living on earth.
- Circular relationships are between elements that act on each other.

Humans look up to the heavens and down to earth, and they look sideways at all the other creatures and objects that exist upon the earth. Together all things move in cycles and circles, including the seasons, the years and the Five Phases (the relationships between earth, fire, metal, water and wood; see chapter 16).

Everything is connected, whether vertically, horizontally or in a cycle.

THE FLOW FROM HEAVEN

The term *jing* (經) denotes the flow of universal life force from heaven to the physical world. This character can also be used for the movement of energy through the meridians in the body in Chinese medicine. The body is like a map of heaven – just as heaven has 12 stems, the body has 12 main meridians and energy flows through them. This reinforces the idea that the world and human existence are built on a constant flow of *chi*.

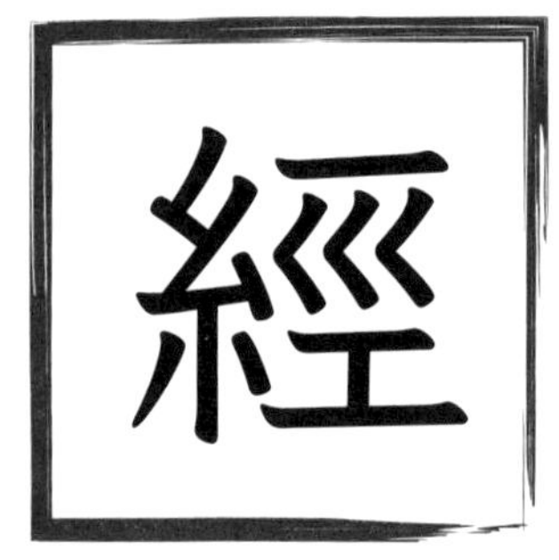

ABOVE:
The character for *jing*.

The network of meridians in the human body are a microcosm of the channels transferring energy between heaven and the physical world.

WORKING WITH YINYANG:
Watch the ebb and flow of energy

When you go into the countryside, take a position where you can see the land for miles around. Notice how the sun moves across the landscape, see which places are always in shadow and which places are always in the sun. If you observe for long enough, through the day, you will notice the movement of yinyang and shake off any notion of a static world.

Then, when you have got used to observing the world as a living, moving system, remember that each entity has its own unique mix of yin and yang and that *chi* flows through all things. Know that you are a part of that, too. When death comes you will divide into the two forms of *chi* and move both upward and downward.

Sense the three relationships: your connection to the sky and to the earth; your place in your surroundings; and your position in the cycles and rhythms that regulate all existence. Energy is not constant, but flows back and forth like the tide.

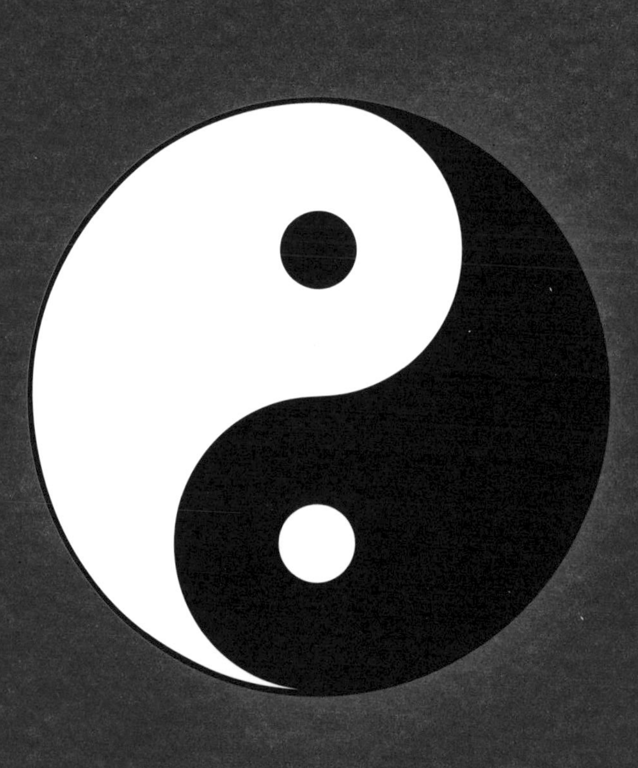

CHAPTER 2

THE ORDER OF THE ANCIENT WORLD

THE ORDER OF THE ANCIENT WORLD

The next step in understanding yinyang is, quite literally, to get your bearings. In old China there were multiple ways of seeing the world, some of which were markedly different from the modern point of view. This chapter will explore those ways. Challenging our own ingrained conception gives us a valuable insight into the ancient Chinese world view.

THE CARDINAL POINTS

On many ancient maps, the south is at the top. This probably has something to do with the spiritual pre-eminence of the sun in ancient times, coupled with the fact that most ancient civilizations, including China, were in the northern hemisphere. In the northern hemisphere, you have to face south in order to trace the movement of the sun across the sky from east to west. Therefore, it made sense to put the south at the top of the map. Indeed, it has only been in the past five hundred years that maps have become standardized with the north at the top.

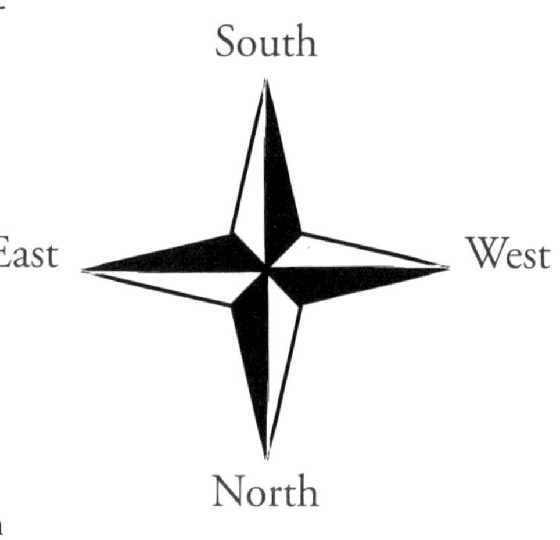

ABOVE RIGHT: Turning the compass upside down is disorientating, but it helps us to understand how the ancient Chinese viewed the world.

The ancient civilizations of the northern hemisphere conceived of the world with south at the top. This is the direction they faced to observe the sun moving across the sky.

THE CARDINAL POINTS AND THE WEATHER

As the ancient Chinese looked about the face of the earth, they perceived that different kinds of weather came from different directions. Some of these are easy to understand; others are not so obvious. Each direction is also associated with one of the Five Phases, the relationships between earth, fire, metal, water and wood, which will be discussed in depth in chapter 16. The table below summarizes these associations.

DIRECTION	WEATHER	PHASE
East	The wind blows from the east.	Wood
South	The heat of the sun comes from the south.	Fire
West	Dryness comes from the west.	Metal
North	Coldness comes from the north because it is away from the sun.	Water
Centre	Dampness comes from the centre.	Earth

☯ **Each point of the compass is connected to a particular type of weather and one of the Five Phases (earth, fire, metal, water and wood).**

THE SIX MEETING DIRECTIONS

The six meeting directions comprise north, south, east and west, and above and below. They meet at a single point in the centre. This is an early Chinese representation of a three-dimensional world view with a human at the centre.

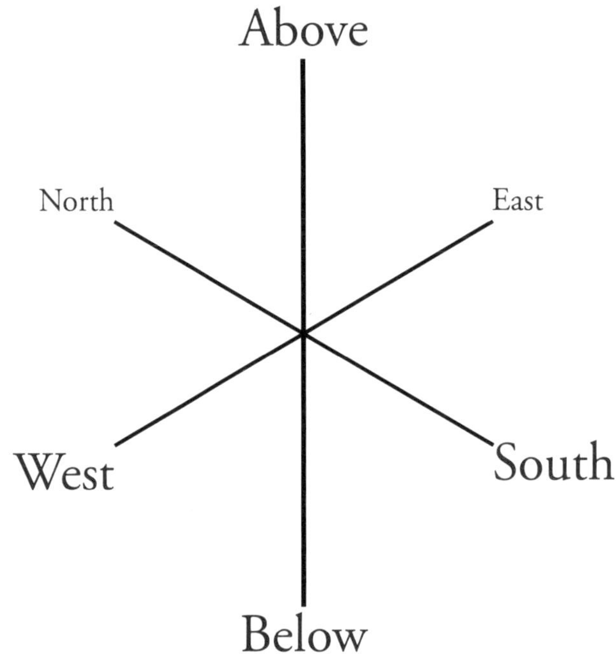

ABOVE: The six meeting directions.

☯ **The six directions of north, south, east, west, above and below meeting at a single point represent a human perspective of the world.**

THE EIGHT OUTWARD DIRECTIONS

The eight directions are a two-dimensional way of representing the world. It is thought that in ancient China the whole land was divided into nine parts: eight squares surrounding a ninth square in the middle. This was also used as a way to organize farmland: the central ninth field contained a well, which served as the water source for the families that farmed the surrounding eight fields. Therefore, the ideogram used in China for a well is a nine-square grid.

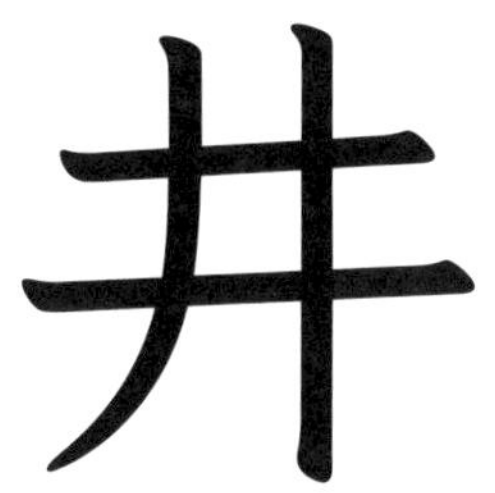

ABOVE: The ideogram for a well.

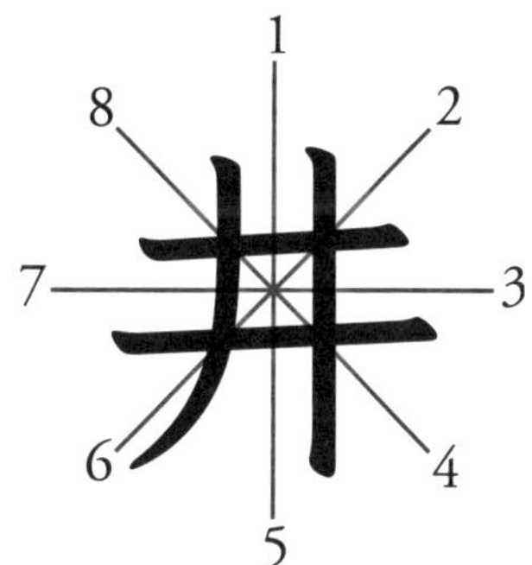

ABOVE: Here each of the eight fields is considered as a direction.

This system encapsulated the idea of looking outward in eight directions. Each of the outer squares represents a direction upon the horizon. This can be seen in the diagram to the right.

The idea of nine squares within a square occurs in numerology, and nine is the highest yang number. This three-by-three grid arrangement became popular in the form of magic squares, where the numbers in each row and column add up to the same total.

The number nine is also significant in relation to the human pulse, which is broken down into nine variations: three pulses in the upper part, three pulses in the middle part and three pulses in the lower part. These are known as the nine territories.

☯ The eight outward directions represented by a three-by-three grid is a key concept in ancient Chinese culture and thought, influencing areas such as farming, numerology and medicine.

THE 12 DIRECTIONS

Building on the six basic directions and the eight field directions is the system of the 12 directions, in which each direction is represented by a different animal. The 12 animal directions and their approximate equivalents on the western compass are given below; a fuller table giving further information can be found on pages 154.

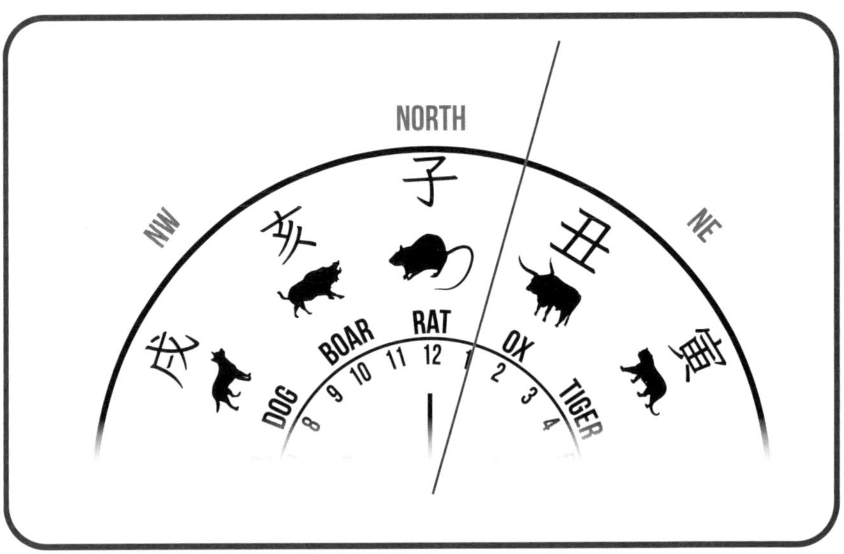

ABOVE: The more complex system of 12 animals became known as the 12 Earthly Branches.

By combining neighbouring directions, it is possible to divide the horizon into 24 directions. For example, the point between the direction of the Rat (north) and the direction of the Ox (approximately northeast by north) can be defined as Rat-Ox (approximately north, northeast).

The number 12 was clearly not plucked from the air, as it relates to the 12 meridians in the human body, the 12 rhythms, the 12 months (although sometimes there are 13 months) and the 12 articulations of the body.

ANIMAL	APPROXIMATE DIRECTION
Rat	North
Ox	NEbN
Tiger	NEbE
Hare	East
Dragon	SEbE
Snake	SEbS
Horse	South
Ram	SWbS
Monkey	SWbW
Cockerel	West
Dog	NWbW
Boar	NWbN

☯ **The 12 directions, each represented by an animal, allow for more precise division of the horizon than the eight outward directions.**

COMPARING THE 12 DIRECTIONS TO THE WESTERN COMPASS

There are 30 degrees between each of the original 12 animals and 15 degrees between each of the directions on the expanded 24-point compass. However, there are 11.25 degrees between each direction on the 32-point western compass, which is why the equivalent directions do not correspond exactly. For example, the direction of the Ox rests at 30 degrees, but the closest cardinal point is northeast by north, which is at 33.75 degrees.

THE DIRECTIONS OF YINYANG BASED ON THE SUN

As in all regions of the northern hemisphere, when you are in China you face south to see the sun pass from east to west. This also means that all shadows created by the sun are cast toward the north. This factor is very important in understanding the idea of yinyang, because the sun is the originator of yinyang theory and dictates which directions are yin and which are yang.

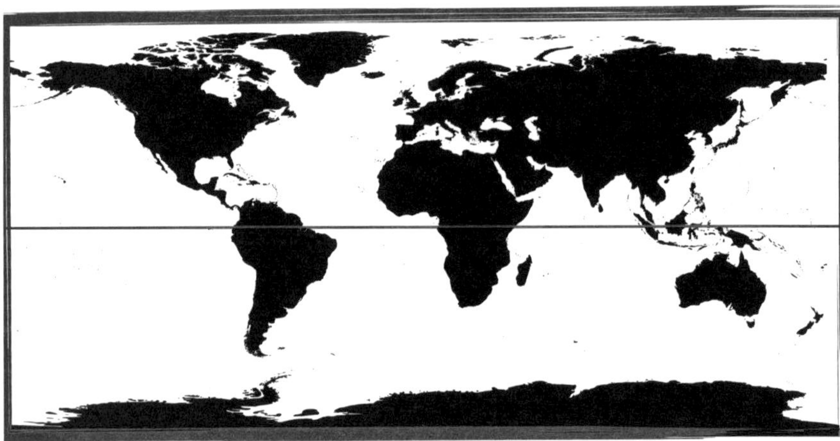

ABOVE: If you live in the northern hemisphere (above the line in this drawing), you can follow many yinyang teachings without a problem. If you live in the southern hemisphere, you may have to reverse some aspects.

To understand this from a human point of view, consider the following points. As you read through them, picture yourself standing in the landscape while the sun travels across the sky.

UP IS YANG

The sun rises as it grows in power each day, reaching its zenith at noon. Therefore, the upward direction is considered to be yang.

LEFT IS YANG

When you face south to observe the sun rising from the east, the east is to your left. Therefore, the left is considered to be yang. This also applies to the left side of the body. This concept only makes sense if you let go of the idea that north is at the top. Turn around and put south at the top instead.

DOWN IS YIN

Yin is down because the sun goes down as it diminishes in power after it has passed the zenith. Therefore, the downward direction is considered to be yin.

RIGHT IS YIN

When you face south to observe the sun setting in the west, the west is to your right. Therefore, the right is considered to be yin. This also applies to the right side of the body.

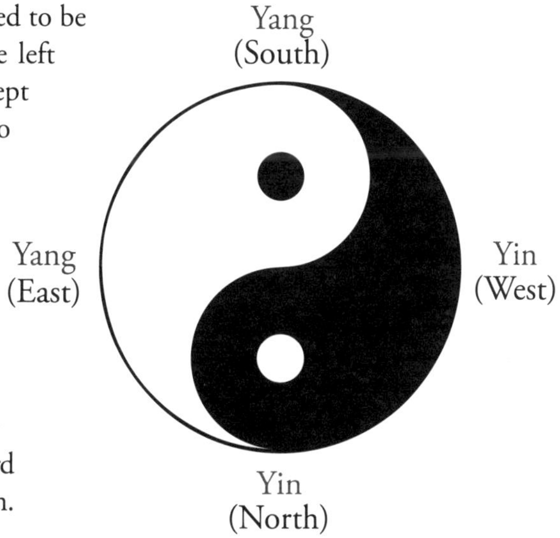

ABOVE: The yinyang symbol itself represents the movement of the sun. The white yang side of the symbol rises up from the left/east like the sun, while the black yin part reaches down to the right/west just as the setting sun does.

The sun's passage across the sky governs which directions are yang and which are yin. Upward and left are yang; downward and right are yin. Anything in sunlight is yang and anything in shadow is yin.

THE DIRECTIONS OF YINYANG BASED ON THE 12 DIRECTIONS

It is important to note here that there is an alternative version of the yinyang directions that derives from the 12 directions instead of the sun. According to this, north and south are yang and east and west are yin.

Remember, the horizon is traditionally divided into 12 sections, and each one is represented by an animal. These animals are associated with either yin or yang. Six animals are yin and six animals are yang, and they alternate between the two as seen in the image below. The animals associated with north and south are both yang; the ones associated with east and west are yin.

This system is used in many ways, including the art of discovering lucky and unlucky days.

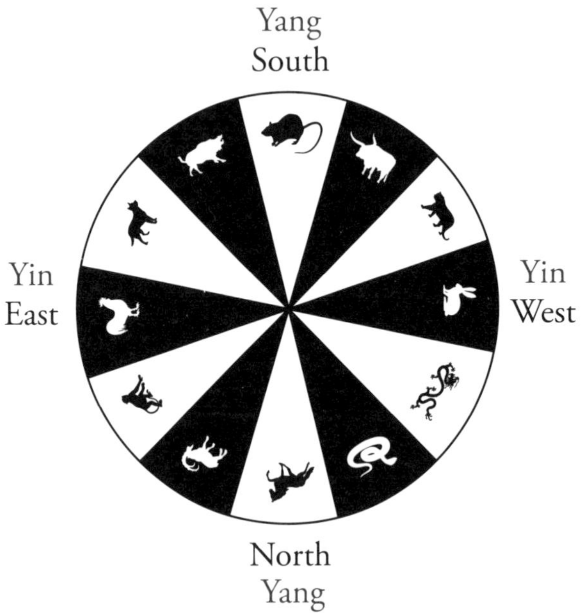

ABOVE: The animal directions alternate between yin and yang.

According to an alternative system based on the 12 directions, north and south are yang and east and west are yin.

THE CIRCLE AND THE SQUARE

Yin earth is represented by a square, while yang sky is a circle. The best way to understand this is that mother earth holds within her all the angular shapes of the ground, while father sky is a dome above the earth containing all the stars.

Still, this can be confusing. The earth is a globe, so why is it represented by a square? Remember, though, that only modern people have seen images of the earth from space. For ancient people, the world was a jagged, rugged place. Think also of the expression "to search the four corners of the world".

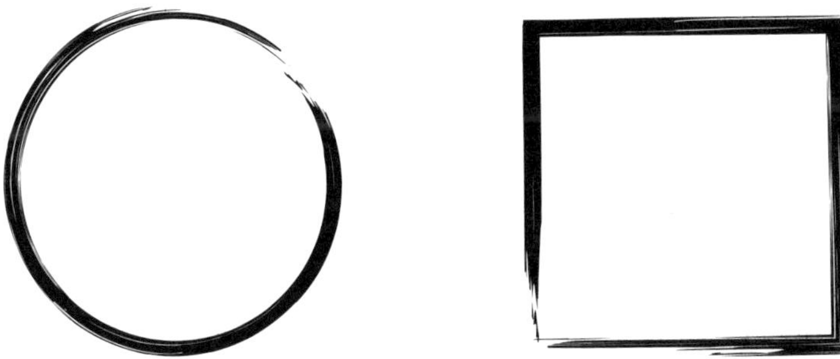

ABOVE: The circle and the square, representing the yang sky and the yin earth respectively.

An ancient text says that a mirror is a circle (yang) and it can be used to reflect the sun and create fire (yang), but when a geometric earthenware pot (yin) is left out in the moonlight, droplets of dew and moisture (yin) form upon it.

☯ **There are no angles in the sky, only on earth. Therefore, the square is a fitting emblem for the angular nature of the physical world. The circle represents the infinite expanse of the sky and the dome of the stars.**

THE ANIMAL KINGDOM

Each species is either yin or yang, but within each species the female is yin and the male is yang. There are two specific animals that are used to represent yin and yang generally: the mare symbolizes female yin energy, while the dragon symbolizes male yang energy. You may often see these two motifs.

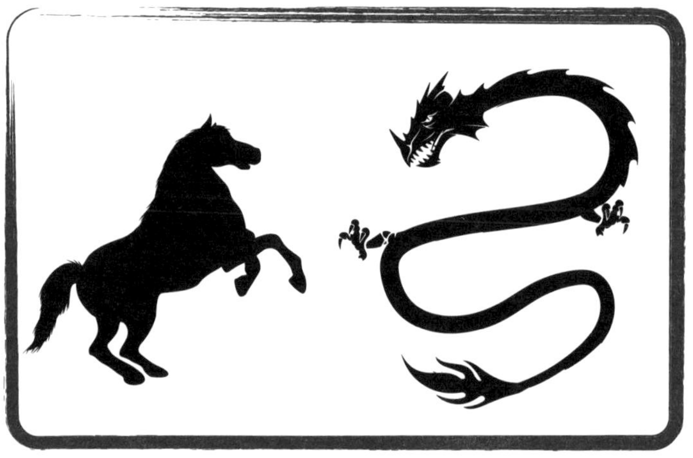

ABOVE: The mare and the dragon, symbols of female yin energy and male yang energy respectively.

Certain principles dictate whether a species is yin or yang. For example, flying creatures with feathers are of the yang aspect, because they can move away from the earth just as yang energy radiates upward into the sky. Fireflies are doubly yang – not only do they fly up into the sky but they also emit light. On the other hand, creatures with scales and shells are of the yin aspect, because they predominantly stay on the ground.

In summer, many animals shed their fur and stags shed their antlers. This is a yang process. Animals that are affected by the movement of the moon are considered to be creatures of yin. For example, fish move down into deeper water during certain phases of the lunar cycle.

All in all, the ancient Chinese saw the world above them as yang, the world around them as yin, the mountains as yang and the valleys as yin, the creatures in the sky as yang and the creatures that dig down as yin.

☯ **The whole of the animal kingdom can be divided into yin and yang creatures, and then each species is subdivided into yin and yang according to its gender.**

WORKING WITH YINYANG:

See yourself as the centre of the universe

We are used to thinking of the world as a globe on which we are each just a tiny and randomly placed dot. In contrast, ancient peoples would have seen themselves as the centre of the universe, the point through which yinyang flows. The ancient Chinese presented the earth in conceptual terms as a square, representing the angles they found around them, and they divided the horizon into sections, each one represented by one of the 12 symbolic animals. Leave your modern mindset behind and try seeing your surroundings in the ancient way. Place yourself back at the centre of the universe; if you move, the universe moves with you. Look in all directions – how does the earth appear to you? Remember that you are at the centre of your world and that you need to navigate the yin and yang that flows through you.

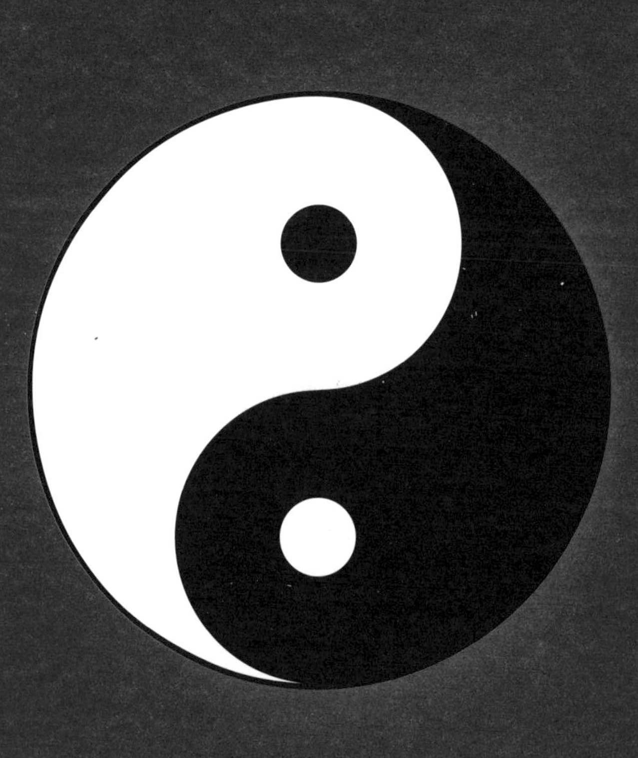

CHAPTER 3

OVERCOMING MISCONCEPTIONS

OVERCOMING MISCONCEPTIONS

We all come to the study of yinyang with certain preconceived ideas, which can hinder our quest to develop a true understanding of the subject. This chapter will remove any misconceptions that may be in your mind, leaving a clear path ahead.

THERE IS NOT ALWAYS BALANCE

Do not fall into the mistake of thinking that yin and yang are always in balance. If you look at the world as a whole, then, yes, it is true that it maintains a natural balance over time: predator–prey relationships, the growth and death of plant life, the changing of the seasons, all are in perfect balance from a cosmic perspective.

However, if you were to stand in the middle of the desert with no shelter in the height of summer, you would suffer from an excess of yang. Likewise, if you were to find yourself standing naked at the North Pole in the darkest point of winter, you would have too much yin. The fact that summer and winter, deserts and ice ranges, are globally in balance does nothing to help the poor person who is burning or freezing to death. These may be extreme examples, but the principle holds true.

Yinyang theory involves riding the waves of change between yin and yang to your best advantage. Put yourself in the right place at the right time doing the right thing to benefit from whichever of the two is predominant.

☯ **Yin and yang balance out over time, but they are rarely in balance at any given moment within a person or a place. Understanding this and acting accordingly will enable you to harness the benefits of yinyang.**

WHERE IS YINYANG?

Heaven is above, the earth is below and humans are in between. Yinyang exists in and around them. Yin accumulates around the surface of the earth, yang descends from the sky and together they mix within the human world. However, although you can see the effects of yinyang by looking at the areas of sun and shade on a mountainside and you can feel heat or moisture in the air, yinyang itself does not manifest physically. It is there between the sky, the earth and humans, but it is not there. So the answer to the question, "Where is yinyang?" is that it was at the beginning of time, it will be at the end of time, it is above you, it is below you and its mixture makes you, it is the all-flowing force that binds the universe.

☯ **Yin and yang meet between heaven and earth where humans live out their lives.**

A BLANKET OF YIN

The very nature of yang chi *is to move outward, while yin* chi *moves downward or inward depending on the context. However, when yang* chi *falls from the sky and mixes with yin* chi *around the earth it appears that the yin* chi *is rising up from the earth, which would directly contradict its natural downward movement. Instead imagine yin* chi *building up around the earth, forming a blanket into which yang* chi *falls from above. This blanket is the layer where the* chi *of heaven, earth and humans mix together. Keep this idea in mind when trying to understand the movement of the* chi *of earth.*

WHAT IS YINYANG?

Yinyang is not a physical thing; it is a state, a way and an idea to be interacted with. On the most basic level it is a set of opposites such as dark and light, cold and hot, small and large. It is a force that helps create the universe and it represents flow from one extreme to the other. Yinyang presents a set of rules that can be followed and a concept that has been studied for thousands of years.

One way to visualize yinyang is as the fabric of the universe, spread out over all time. In cloth making, the parallel strands stretched out separately on the loom are called the warp, while the thread woven between them is called the weft. Yinyang binds together with the four seasons like this to create the fabric of reality in which humans live.

An ancient text from China says the following:

- Heaven is the father.
- Earth is the mother.
- Yinyang is the warp of the fabric of reality.
- The four seasons are the weft of the fabric of reality.

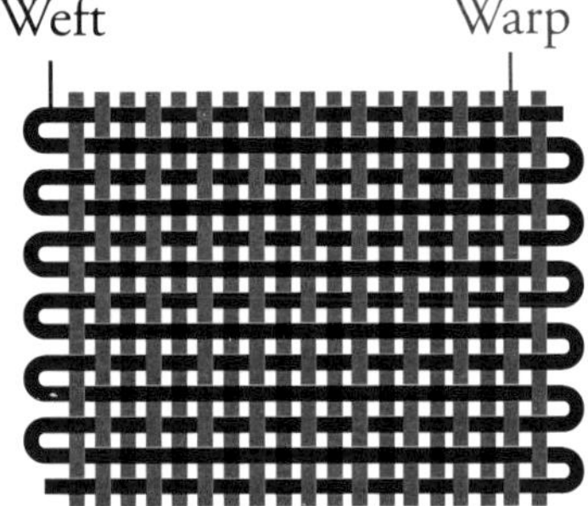

ABOVE: Yinyang is the fabric of reality, the material that binds all life together in a living tapestry.

Heaven, earth and the four seasons are phenomena that humans can see or experience, but yinyang is the binding thread that connects everything.

☯ **Yinyang is a state not a physical entity. It is the pattern that holds reality in place.**

TYPES OF ENERGY

Yang energy by nature expands and moves outward, it seeks to disperse and radiate. Yin energy tends to retract, come together and congeal. For example, the yang energy of the body radiates outward during the day but at night yin takes over and pulls all energy back into the body so that it can sleep and recuperate. The sun is yang and it bursts with energy, whereas the moon is yin and it absorbs or reflects the sun's radiance, rather than shining with its own light.

☯ **Yang radiates, yin contracts. This is the nature of yin and yang *chi*.**

HUMAN INFLUENCE ON YINYANG

While the ancient Chinese viewed yinyang as a universal law, they also believed that their behaviour could affect the balance of yinyang for better or worse. This happened as a result of human *chi* energy radiating outward and mingling with cosmic *chi*, like ripples from a pebble that has been dropped into the water. Too big a splash could throw yinyang out of balance.

Natural disasters such as whirlwinds, droughts, floods and plagues were seen as retribution for human cruelty or unjust punishments. Daoist masters observed omens and portents, and if they detected a harmful imbalance of yinyang they would instruct the people to perform certain rituals and actions to make sure the *chi* from the community was in accordance with the *chi* of the universe.

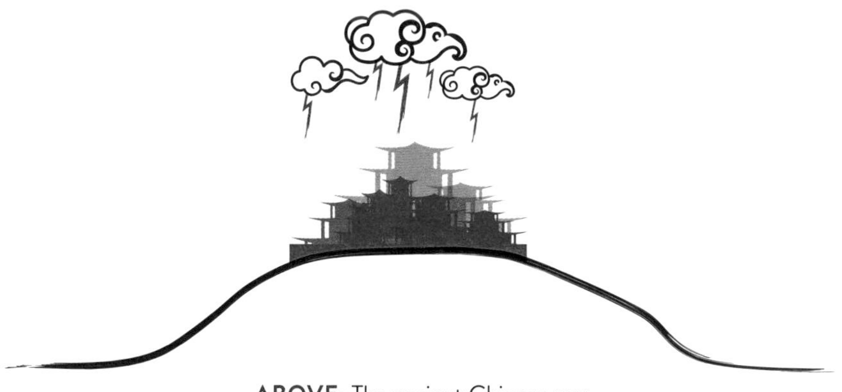

ABOVE: The ancient Chinese saw extreme weather events as the result of human *chi* affecting the balance of yinyang.

This is a far-reaching issue which harks back to the basic questions of human existence. Who or what created us and why? Is there a purpose to existence? Can we interact with this purpose? Is anyone or anything out there listening to us? For the Chinese that something was the Dao, but none of us can know what it is for sure.

☯ Human behaviour can disrupt the balance of yinyang. In ancient times the population looked to Daoist masters to restore order through ritual and action.

THE ANCIENT CHINESE CALENDAR

The Chinese calendar differs greatly from the modern western calendar. Whereas the western New Year always falls on 1 January, Chinese New Year changes its date depending on the calculations for that year. The year itself is divided into either 12 or 13 months based on a relationship between the sun, the moon and the stars. Months are known as large months or small months and extra days have to be inserted at times to keep the calendar aligned. There are 12 zodiac signs, including Monkey, Dog, Horse and so on, which give their names to the hours, days, months and years. The 12 zodiac signs combine with the Five Phases (see chapter 16) to create a 60-year cycle of year names. Each year within the cycle has certain meanings, to which the Chinese pay close attention.

In ancient China the day was divided into 12 hours, each one approximately 120 minutes long. There were six hours during the daytime and six hours during the night. However, the hours would actually shorten and lengthen according to the times of sunrise and sunset (this no longer happens in modern Asia). It is important to be aware of the workings of the Chinese calendar when you study aspects of yinyang that relate to time.

☯ **The Chinese calendar system has a cycle of 60 years and the hours, days, months and years are all represented by animals. The ancient Chinese day had 12 hours, six in the daylight and six at night.**

YINYANG ASSOCIATIONS

Yin and yang have certain contrasting associations. Something is either of the yin aspect or the yang aspect, but that status can change depending on the context (see the next point). The following table gives an overview of yinyang associations.

YINYANG ASSOCIATIONS	
YIN	YANG
Negative	Positive
Static	Dynamic
Female	Male
Moon	Sun
Autumn	Spring
Winter	Summer
Square	Circle
Earth	Heaven / Sky
Water	Fire
West	East
North	South
Night	Day
Dark	Light
Down	Up
Right	Left
Internal	External
Non-movement	Movement

YINYANG ASSOCIATIONS	
YIN	YANG
Even numbers	Odd numbers
Music	Dancing
Descending	Ascending
Solid	Liquid, vapour or gas
Soft	Hard
Cold	Hot
Dim	Bright
Material component	Functionality or nature

Remember that in some schools east and west are yin and north and south are yang.

☯ **Fire and water were created at the same time and they come from the same origin point, but one turns into yin and the other turns into yang.**

YIN AND YANG IN RELATION TO EACH OTHER

Not all the yinyang associations listed in the previous table are constant. Some may change according to context. For example, a cup of boiling hot tea is yang compared to a cup of warm tea, which in this case is yin. However, if the cup of warm tea is put next to a cup of ice tea, the warm tea becomes yang and the ice tea is yin.

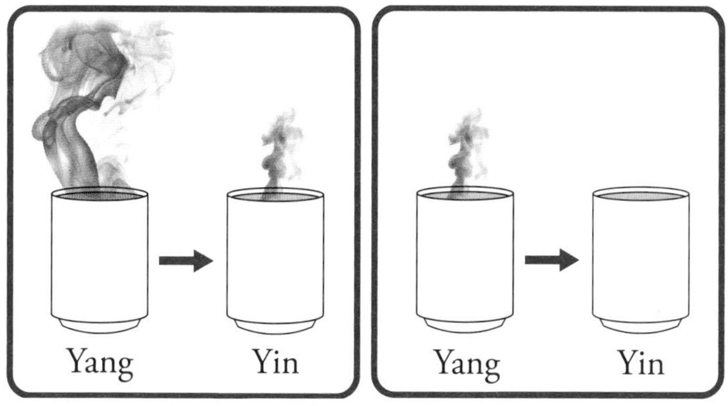

ABOVE: Warm tea is yin compared to boiling hot tea, but yang compared to ice tea.

The following table itemizes some of the principal yinyang relationships.

YINYANG RELATIONSHIPS	
YIN	YANG
Colder	Hotter
Softer	Harder
Weaker	Stronger
Lower	Higher
Smaller	Larger
Shorter	Longer

The yin or yang quality of everything in the universe can change in comparison with something else.

YINYANG IN ACTION

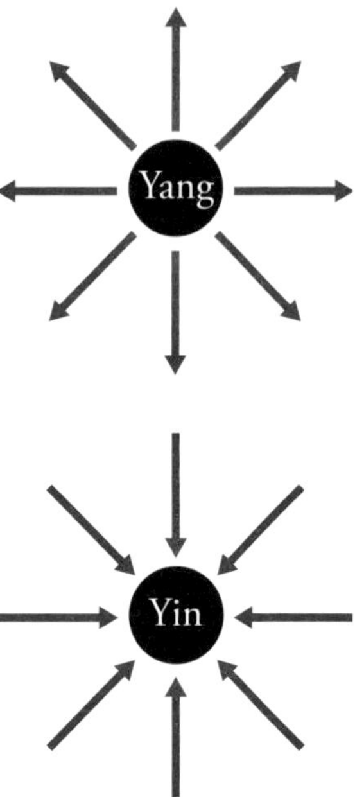

Yang is to go outward, yin is to move inward; yang is to stretch outward, yin is to bend; yang is to extend, yin is to contract. Of course, context can affect this – something that goes out a little way is yin compared to something that goes out a long way – but overall yang is outward movement, yin is inward movement.

RIGHT: Yang expands, yin contracts.

Outward movement is yang, inward movement is yin. This is a fundamental principle of yinyang.

A SHIFTING RELATIONSHIP

It can be said that yin and yang do not exist except in relation to each other. When the first people called the sunshine on a hillside "yang" and the shade "yin" they created a relationship between two states. When the sun moved, the areas of shadow and light moved too, and so did the relationship. From this basic idea developed a complex system of relationships that spilt into many schools of thought. From the movements of the planets to the workings of *chi* in the human body, the universe is not static and neither is yinyang. It all depends on how things are observed.

Yinyang relationships are not static.

HEAVENLY PROTECTION

Something can be yang in itself, but have a yin relationship with something else. For example, the sky is yang, but the blanket of air it creates to envelop the earth is yin (as yin is associated with cover and protection). In the same way, the shade a tree casts on the ground is yin while the tree itself is yang.

DUALISTIC BUT NOT ANTAGONISTIC

When speaking of yinyang, the terms "dualism" and "duality" often come up. It is true that yinyang is a dualistic concept involving the relationship between opposites. However, that does not mean yin and yang *oppose* each other. They coexist in harmony and do not attack their opposite or try to wipe it out. A reduction of one element will mean a rise in the other, but they are not at war with each other.

☯ **Yinyang is like pouring water back and forth between two jugs. The total amount of water never changes, but at times one jug may be empty while the other is full.**

WORKING WITH YINYANG:

Know that yinyang shapes your life

There will be times when your situation is extremely yang and other times when it is extremely yin. Yinyang is everywhere at all times and it is the foundation of the realm in which we exist. You are forever in a relationship with the landscape and the skyscape, and this relationship is continually changing as you move within your existence. Your actions can affect the balance of yinyang, and yinyang can affect you. Remember that yin and yang are not at war with each other – and they are not at war with you. It is just that being in the wrong place at the wrong time can mean you are overwhelmed by either one. In the simplest of terms: if you stand at the North Pole with no clothes, you will freeze; if you wear a fur coat in the desert, you will swelter. Try to understand and read the signs of yinyang so you can move in harmony with it and ride the waves of transformation.

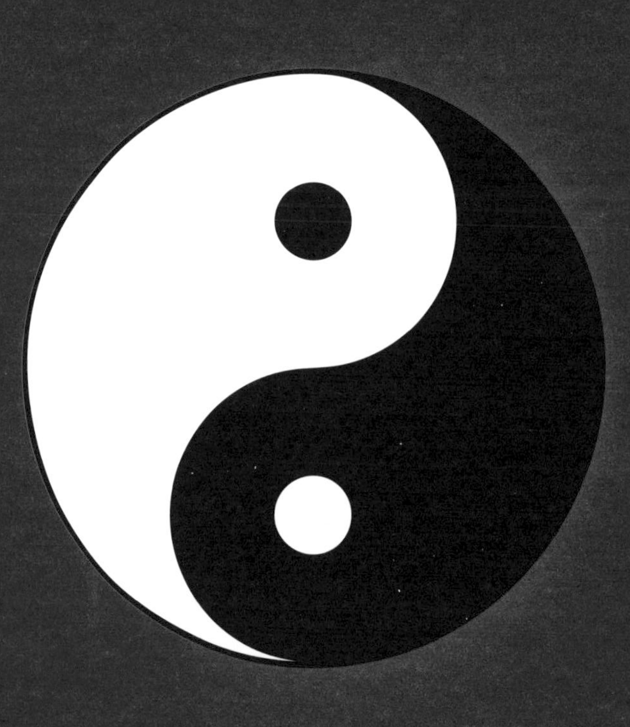

CHAPTER 4

YINYANG IN MOTION

YINYANG IN MOTION

Now you have gained a basic understanding of yinyang, it is time to see how the process moves, how it lives. This chapter will smash through any last boundaries that remain within your mind, helping you to move from the idea of yin and yang as opposite forces to a picture of yinyang in constant motion, a swirling of both sides as they mix together to create a dynamic whole.

USING ANALOGY

If you have read the Dao De Jing by Lao Tzu you will be familiar with the statement, "The Way is indescribable and if you can describe it then it is not the true Way." This famous saying is referring to the Dao, but it applies equally to yinyang. The building blocks of the universe are beyond human understanding, but that does not mean we cannot *try* to comprehend them. The ancient Chinese often used analogy to convey such indiscernible concepts. The following are some examples that have been used to help people grasp the fluidity of yinyang.

THE TREE

In this analogy, the roots represent yinyang. Hidden underground, the roots sustain all other parts of the tree. Every single leaf on every single twig of every single branch owes its existence to the roots. Just like the roots of a tree, yinyang reaches into the world and affects all things.

Beyond this basic meaning, the tree can also be divided into aspects of yinyang that change depending on how they are viewed:

- The tree itself is yang; the shadow it casts is yin.
- The parts above ground are yang; those below ground are yin.
- The trunk is yang; the branches are yin.
- The branches are yang; the leaves are yin.
- The upper part of the leaf is yang; the underside is yin.

Note that the branches are yin in relation to the trunk, but yang in relation to the leaves.

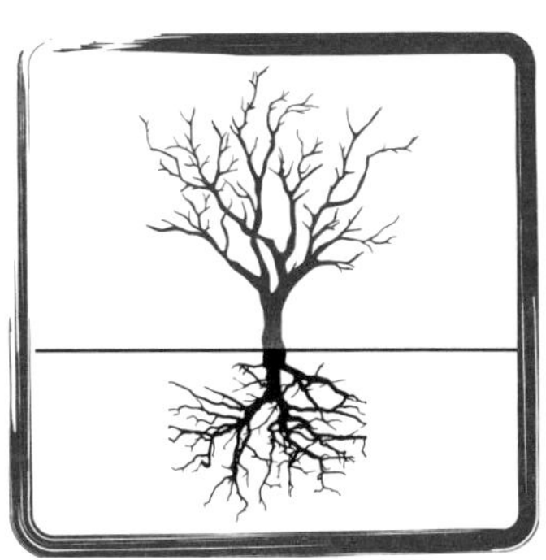

ABOVE: Yinyang is the root of existence, feeding all other parts of the tree of life.

The tree analogy relates to an important eastern concept known as the "origin and the periphery" (本末), literally "trunk and branches". Knowing that all things have a centre and external points helps people make sense of their experience of life. This theory is known in Chinese as *benmo* and in Japanese as *honmatsu*.

BENMO* AND *HONMATSU				
IDEOGRAM	TRANSLATION	MEANING	CHINESE	JAPANESE
本	trunk	origin / centre	*ben*	*hon*
末	branches	periphery	*mo*	*matsu*

All actions originate in intentions from a core element. Crops come from seeds planted in fields; when the land dries out it is because the sun was too hot, and when it floods it is because there was too much rain. Love starts within the mind but is projected outwardly; combat and bloodshed are the result of desire or anger; and the greatest cities of the world are the result of human ingenuity.

All of these examples show how the origin creates the effect and how nothing exists without a starting point. The origin and periphery theory underpins much of yinyang and Traditional Chinese Medicine.

☯ **All things have an origin and yinyang is at the root of everything.**

THE DOOR

Another way to understand yinyang is as a door. Imagine a door set in a wall. If the door is permanently secured either open or closed, it is no longer a door. If it is always open, it becomes nothing more than a passageway. If it is always closed, it is only part of a wall. In either case, the door has ceased to function as a door. The nature of a door is that it can change from being open to closed and back again. It is the same with yinyang, which by its very nature is always moving from one state to the other. If everything were always yang or always yin, there would be no movement and no universe.

Yinyang can either help or hinder your plans depending on timing. The same is true of a door. If the door is locked when you want to pass through or wedged open when you want to stop other people getting in or out, this tells you that you are trying to do the wrong thing at the wrong time. Yinyang is constantly in flux and we must learn its rhythms.

☯ **Yinyang sometimes lets us pass and sometimes blocks our way, sometimes protects us and sometimes exposes us. We have to read its rhythms and time our movements accordingly.**

THE WHEEL

If a cart wheel is too rigid it will snap on a bumpy road; too flexible and it will wear away quickly. By combining layers of soft and strong wood, ancient wheelwrights were able to produce a durable wheel that still had enough flexibility to adapt to the surface of the road. This is how yinyang works – two contrasting qualities mixed together to create perfection.

☯ **Everything, no matter what its nature, is a combination of yin and yang.**

THE RIVER

When the universe was created, did all yinyang come into being at that moment or is yinyang continually creating itself and the universe over time? The best way to approach this question is to forget about creation points like the so-called Big Bang, and focus more on the *flow* of yinyang. Just as you cannot step into the same river twice because the water is always flowing, yinyang is constantly transforming. Physical reality is in a state of continuous flux as the source of all life streams through it. You are not looking for a start point, nor are you looking for an end; what matters is the place where the river flows, ever changing but ever present – this is yinyang.

Nothing is ever destroyed, only transformed, as yinyang flows through our lives.

POTENTIAL FOR CHANGE

Within yinyang the dominant element at the time always has the potential to change. Yang can become yin because yang has a small element of yin within it, and vice versa. Someone who starts as a good person may go astray, while a thoroughly villainous character may become good. This idea is reflected in the famous yinyang symbol, where the black section has some white in it and the white has some black.

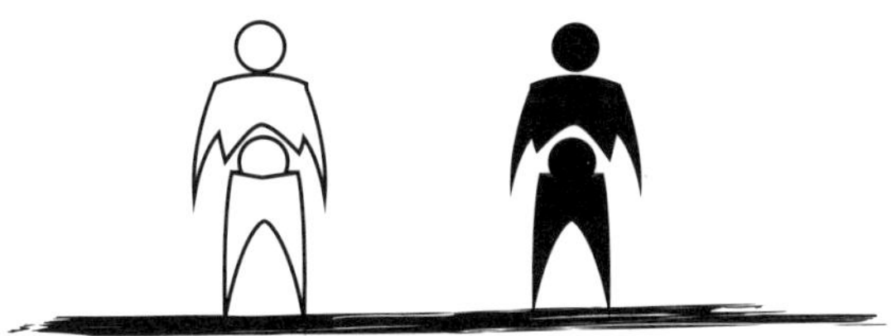

ABOVE: Things can change to their total opposite and then back again. Nothing is ever static.

Yang contains its future state of yin and yin contains its future state of yang.

CHANGE OR REPLACE?

The use of non-Chinese terms such as "change", "transform", "mutate" and "become" to explain how yin and yang move into each other gives rise to certain philosophical questions. Do yin and yang change into each other or do they actually replace each other? Is it new yin (or yang) or is it old yin (or yang) returned? This is all part of the unknowable nature of yinyang.

ASPECTS OF THE WHOLE

Yin and yang are not entirely separate entities. We often see yin as black and yang as white, but they merge into each other to form a single universe with two polar opposites and a full scale of shades in between. If something is yang it will eventually move toward yin and if it is yin it will eventually move toward yang. If there is an imbalance, such as a drought or a flood, or if a person is cold or has a fever, then balance needs to be restored. At times of drought there is too much yang (heat) in the world, so in old China they would engage in yin activities to bring about yin *chi*. Whereas if there is too much rain – which is yin – then yang aspects would be focused on to promote yang *chi* to dry up the excess water.

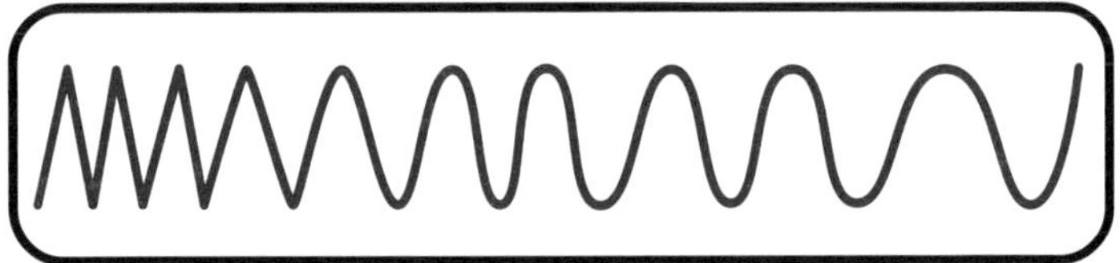

ABOVE: Think of yinyang as an energy wave where the frequency oscillates between two extremes.

If something is too yin, then either yin needs to be taken away or yang needs to be added. If there is too much yang, then either yang needs to be taken away or yin needs to be added.

ONE WITHIN THE OTHER

While yin and yang are born from each other and are not separate forms, they are still distinguishable from each other to a certain degree. You can have yin inside of yang and yang inside of yin, just like gifts contained within a series of smaller and smaller boxes.

For example, the ground is yin and a seed is also yin. So when a seed is planted in the soil, there is a yin element inside a yin place. However, when the seed germinates it becomes yang. The rising force of the plant is a yang power within the yin quietness of the soil.

Likewise, the brightness of day is yang, while the darkness of night is yin. The morning with its dawning light is yang, even though it is still on the edge of darkness; while the afternoon, though it is still light, will soon become night and therefore is considered as yin. The first part of the night is yin within yin but as night gets closer to morning then it becomes yang within yin. Just as the day can be divided up into four yinyang sections, so can the year, making a day a microcosm of the year (see table below).

TIME OF DAY	SEASON	DIVISION
Sunrise to noon	Summer	Yang within yang
Noon to dusk	Autumn	Yin within yang
Nightfall to cock's crow	Winter	Yin within yin
Cock's crow to dawn	Spring	Yang within yin

This idea can be taken even further; you can keep subdividing again and again. However, you must always remember what the top layer is so that you know whether you are predominantly within the aspect of yin or of yang.

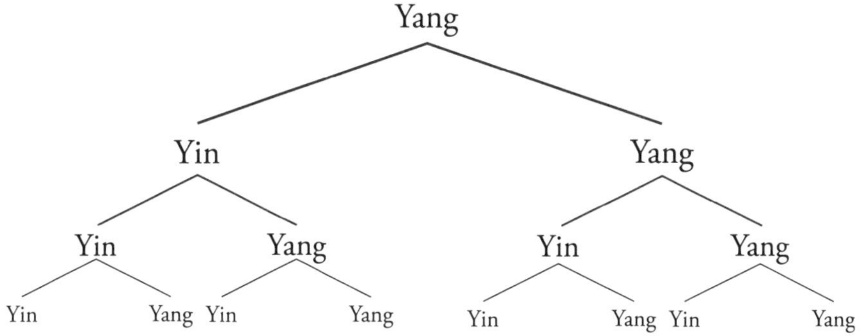

ABOVE: Yin and yang within each other can produce a complex family tree despite having only two members.

The concept of yin within yang and yang within yin was also observed by the ninja of Japan. In his 1676 manual, the *Bansenshukai* (萬川集海), ninja master Fujibayashi Yasutake explains that a ninja spy can infiltrate an enemy fortress either by adopting a disguise and entering in plain sight (yang) or by sneaking about in stealth (yin). However, if a ninja uses a disguise to walk through the first line of defence and then moves in stealth when they get closer to the target, their mission becomes yin within yang. (Fujibayashi-sensei's complete secret scroll has been translated into English as *The Book of Ninja*, published by Watkins.)

THE OBSERVABLE AND THE UNOBSERVABLE

Do not ignore what you cannot see. That which is in power holds something hidden within it that will go on to take control. The soil in winter holds the plants for spring and summer. The darkness of night is on one side of the earth, but the world will turn to reveal the brightness of the sun.

If humans did not know that a seed put into the earth held the promise of a fruiting plant, civilisation would not have gone very far. While observing the observable, always take into account things you cannot see, which may affect you at a later point.

☯ **Yin or yang is hidden within the now, ready to become dominant in the future. One of the benefits of being human is the ability to predict change.**

THE THREE VARIABLES

There are three main factors that can throw yinyang out of balance and bring disharmony to a situation.

- **Speed, known as *jiezou*** (節奏) – this is the idea that yin or yang is too slow or too fast. If it is either one then problems occur and things will need to be slowed down or sped up.

- **Volume, known as *pinghen*** (平衡) – this is the idea that if there is too much yin or too much yang for too long then the opposite element needs increasing so as to decrease the influence of the dominant one.

- **Force, known as *bianhua*** (變化) – this is the idea that the change from yin to yang or yang to yin is too weak or too strong. Efforts to regain harmony may not have been enough or may have gone too far.

☯ To rebalance yinyang, it may be necessary to speed things up or slow things down, increase one element or sap the other, or adjust the force of change. Get these things wrong and there will be struggle ahead.

LAYERS OF COMPLEXITY

Yinyang theory is essentially very simple: yin and yang can be absolute opposites (black and white, hot and cold) or they can be relative opposites (darker and lighter, hotter and colder). It is also quite easy to grasp the idea that yin and yang change into each other in natural processes such as day becoming night and night becoming day. However, yinyang relationships can soon become extremely complex. Alfred Forke (1867–1944), a German scholar of Chinese philosophy, gave the following example to illustrate the problem:

"The left hand is yang while the right hand is yin. When both hands are held above the head they are in a yang position, but if they are lowered by your sides they are in a yin position. If the hands are hot they are yang and if cold they are yin."

Working through Forke's statement, if your left hand is at your side it is a yang hand in a yin position, but if it is hot then it is a yang hand in a yin position with a yang temperature. If the hand becomes cold, it becomes a yang hand in a yin position with a yin temperature. If the cold hand is raised up high, it is a yang hand in a yang position with a yin temperature, and if the hand becomes hot again it will be a yang hand in a yang position with a yang temperature. And we have not even mentioned the right hand yet. This is a simple way of showing how quickly the yinyang relationships in the world can become complex and confusing. If you come across something that appears to be labelled the opposite of what you expected, it will most likely be because of the relationship it has to a vast number of other aspects. These apparent anomalies often occur in Traditional Chinese Medicine, which can become confusing because of the complexity of the body.

☯ **The simple principles of yinyang soon get left behind when a string of factors are viewed in relation to each other. If something is called yin when it looks like it should be yang, we need to think of all the relationships connected to it rather than assuming that it is a mistake.**

SPACE AND STRUCTURE

Consider this old Chinese lesson. Which part of a jug is more important: the clay structure (yang) or the space within it (yin)? The answer is that the empty space is the truly important part of the jug, because this is where the liquid is held. Without the space the jug would not function. The same is true of a house. Take the walls of a house and place them in a line and you no longer have a house. It is the empty space within those walls that makes a house useful.

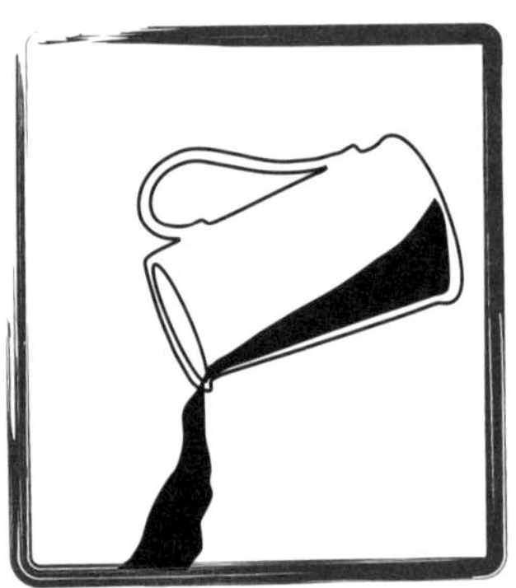

ABOVE: A jug is not a jug without the capacity to hold liquid.

In contrast, the purpose of a spade is to dig and it is the solid yang element of the spade that enables it to function. If you try to dig or shovel with a garden fork, the loose soil will fall through the yin spaces between the yang tines.

Everything has both form and function. It is important to know which aspect of something is more useful: its physical structure or the non-physical space it holds. We should use yin when we need yin, and yang when we need yang.

WORKING WITH YINYANG:
Observe and predict the patterns

Take note of the rising and setting of the sun, the phases of the moon, the changing positions of the stars and the ways the seasons play out in nature. Look at a river and see how the ripples stay in the same position but the water moves through them. All such things are yinyang in motion. Observe the changes in your surroundings and your life, and learn to read the signals of change. Take your observations a step further and start predicting the patterns instead of just watching them. Always remember that you need to work with both yin and yang, so it can be harmful to identify too strongly with one element or the other.

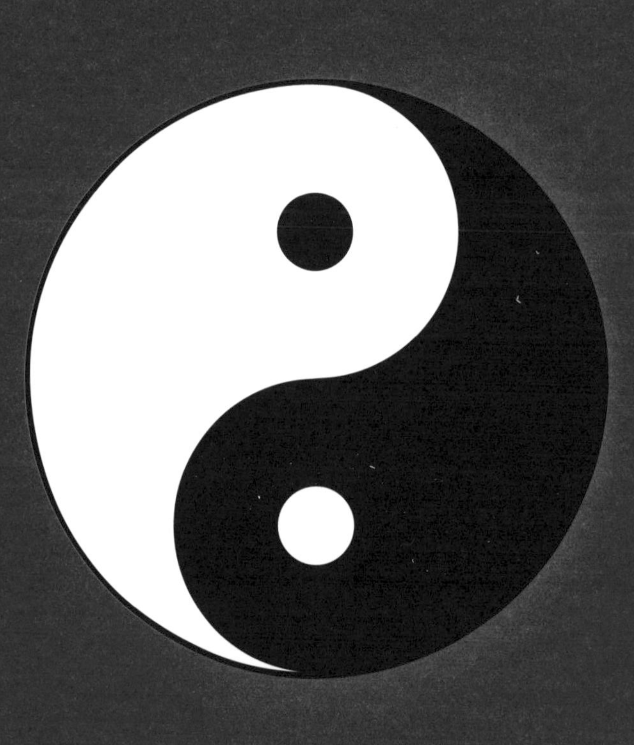

CHAPTER 5

MOVING WITH THE DAO

MOVING WITH THE DAO

To understand yinyang you need to have a grasp of the Dao – the Way. For the ancient Chinese, the Dao was universal, or at least understood by all as a concept, no matter which school of thought they followed, and the term "the Way" even permeated into Buddhism and other eastern cultures. The Dao is a far-reaching idea and is fundamental to the concept of yinyang.

THE DAO IS THE ORIGIN

In ancient Chinese mythology, the Dao or Way is the "thing" behind the creation of the universe. When the universe came into being, the "something" of the pre-universe divided into yin and yang. This movement gave rise to *chi* energy, which was the spark required to create life. Everything emanates from this source. Yinyang acts as a thread that connects all life together, and *chi* animates it.

Therefore, reality is not the sum of all the small parts that exist within it; all those small parts are results of the movement of yinyang. The Dao is in one sense a part of the fabric of reality, but it also exists outside it as the pattern behind the universe.

☯ **While being behind all tangible parts of the universe, the Dao itself is intangible and beyond the realm of human comprehension.**

COSMIC CONSCIOUSNESS

Daoist thought suggests that "consciousness" (for want of a better term) existed before the material world, but that it needed matter to anchor itself within existence – an awkward paradox. This is similar to the theory of Biocentrism formulated by the American scientist Robert Lanza (born 1956), according to which life creates the universe. Lanza argues that physical properties of the universe such as light, colour, temperature and sound owe their existence to being perceived in the consciousness of living beings.

Buddhism says that true reality is outside of our understanding and that we are searching to get back to the state of the Buddha, while Daoism says that reality is in existence because of the principal law which gave birth to the material realm. Humans are just an expression of the principal law and their essence returns to it after death. Therefore, we have to ask the question, "What is the consciousness of the universe and how does that relate to human consciousness?"

WHAT CAN WE KNOW ABOUT THE UNKNOWABLE?

We know the Dao was at the start of all things and is the system behind creation, but beyond that, what do we know about it? For example, does the Dao have consciousness? This question is impossible to answer because it needs to be approached from so many different directions, including the following, each of which is as unknowable as the Dao itself.

- Does the Dao have consciousness on a cosmic level?
- Does the Dao know we exist?
- Does the Dao understand human consciousness?
- Can the Dao read our thoughts?
- Does the Dao involve itself in our lives?
- Do we have a fate or destiny given to us by the Dao?

It is said that the Dao is beyond good and evil, that it has no concept of right or wrong, but it is also often said that a person must be in tune with the Dao to achieve their objectives. Furthermore, the concept of *wuwei*, or non-focused action (see page 301), indicates that the Way provides the best path for those who follow a natural lifestyle – adding to the notion that the Dao is benevolent to an extent.

The Dao is said to be inexhaustible and infinite. If this is so, then why do humans go without? Some say that it is because society has lost touch with the Dao, which implies that there are correct paths to choose, which in turn implies that the Dao has knowledge of human behaviour.

These questions are endless, and volume upon volume has been written with arguments lasting centuries. Yet there are certain points on which most Daoist thinkers have come to agree, including the following:

- The Dao is outside of time and space yet flows through it.
- The Dao created time and space.
- The Dao gives life to everything.
- The Dao works through yinyang movement.
- The Dao is never exhausted.
- The Dao can provide for all life.
- Some lifeforms go unprovided for because they are not in tune with the Dao.
- If the Dao is followed then life is fruitful and easy.

☯ **While the only thing that can be known for certain about the Dao is that it is unknowable, we must conclude that the Dao understands correct behaviour to be positive even if it does not take sides in human affairs.**

THE DAO IS THE CONSTANT

The Dao is the only truly constant thing in the universe. The four seasons follow a predictable cycle, but they still bring changes. The Dao is never seen but never wavers. In mathematical terms, it is the constant equation that keeps the universe in motion.

☯ **The Dao changes everything, yet never changes.**

GENERATION AND TRANSFORMATION

The movement of the universe generates *chi*, and that *chi* creates all things in existence. All things begin as potential beings. They are then generated. After this, they are transformed, and then they die before being re-formed. The cycle is never-ending.

The process is similar to Buddhist reincarnation. The major difference is that Buddhists believe that beings retain elements of their past incarnations, whereas in Daoism *chi* is re-formed and it is not known whether it is influenced at all by its previous forms.

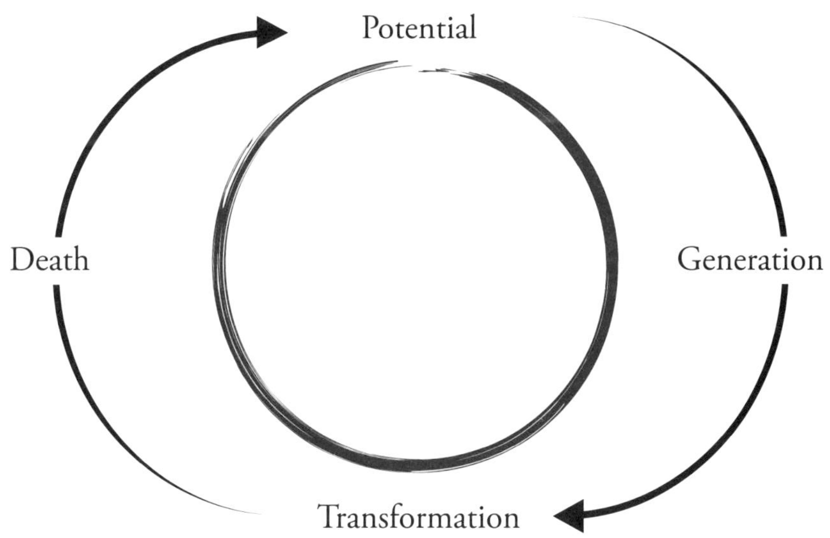

ABOVE: The cycle of existence.

In Daoism, life is cyclical. The stages are: potential, generation, transformation and death. After death *chi* is re-formed into new potential life.

TYPES OF BEING

Within the cycle of life and death, there are two categories of being: constant and regenerative.

CONSTANT BEINGS

The rising and setting of the sun, the phases of the moon, the tides of the ocean, these are all constant. The same sun, the same moon, the same water. They move in cycles, but over time these cycles never change. You can "never bathe in the same river twice", but you are still bathing in water that cannot change its nature and that will always exist somewhere in the world.

REGENERATIVE BEINGS

Humans, fauna, flora, minerals, these are all things that are born and die. New rock is created from the layering of sediment or the heat of the earth, plants set seeds, humans and animals reproduce. While the species continue, they do so through a process of regeneration in which each individual being has a limited life span.

☯ **Even rocks will grind to dust and new mountains form, but water will always be water and fire will always be fire.**

THE UNIVERSE IS A YINYANG MACHINE

The universe is an amazing machine, powered by *chi* and regulated by yinyang. Nothing can ever be added or taken away from the universe; existence is a perpetual process of transformation as yin and yang rise and fall in their untiring rhythm.

There is more than enough *chi* in the universe to sustain all life. Problems only occur when human societies deviate from the Way. We must remember that we are all part of this system. By following the Way, individuals bring benefit to all people in the world.

☯ **The universe is a machine that never stops. The Dao is the law that keeps the machine running.**

WORKING WITH YINYANG:

Move with the Dao

By attuning yourself to the natural rhythms of the world – the shortening and lengthening of days, the growth and decay of plants, the waxing and waning of the moon – you learn how to read and predict the patterns of yinyang. Consider how all these processes relate to each other and picture them as the workings of a single organic machine that never stops running. That machine works in accordance with the Dao – the set of laws that govern all of creation. Your goal is to move with the Dao and it is the goal of this book to teach you how to do that.

Yinyang was born from the Dao. The movement and distribution of yinyang, along with the power of *chi*, created the whole universe. Every moment of every day, the miracle of creation is happening as yin and yang move in and out of dominance. As the *chi* of the earth accumulates and the *chi* of the sky descends, the *chi* of humans mixes within it and can cause an imbalance. By focusing on acts that will generate yin or yang *chi*, we can help restore the balance. See yourself as being on the path of the Dao.

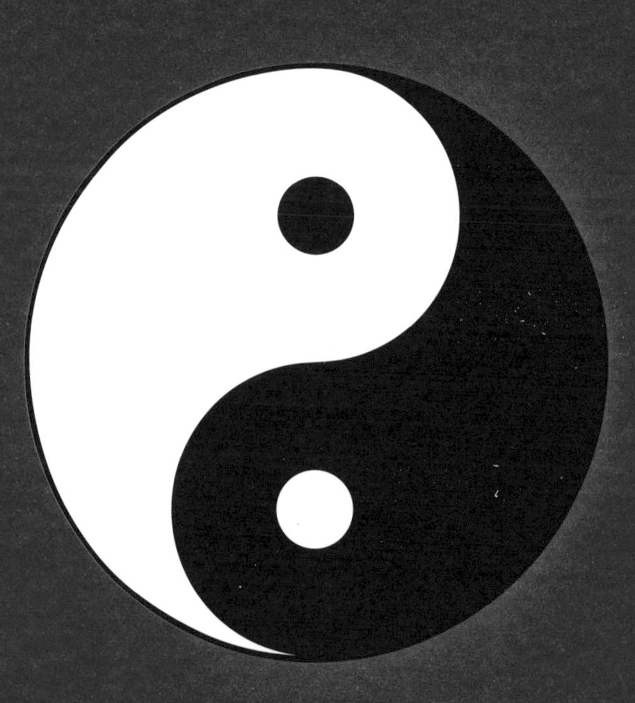

CHAPTER 6

YINYANG AND GENDER

YINYANG AND GENDER

There is a common misconception that yin is female and yang is male. Females are categorized as yin and males are yang, but this does not mean that yin itself is female, nor yang male. It also does not mean that other entities categorized as yin or yang are male or female. The yin moon is not female and the yang sun is not male. They are of no gender. Yinyang relationships are often described in terms of male and female – for example, "father sky and mother earth" – but that is humans projecting gender onto them through linguistic labels. The following chapter addresses issues of gender in the context of yinyang. This will enable you to correct your own misunderstandings and those of other people.

POSITIVE AND NEGATIVE

One problem that needs to be fixed early on is the misunderstanding of positive and negative. In yinyang theory yin is negative and yang is positive, but this does not mean that yin is bad and yang is good, and it certainly does not mean that male (yang) is superior to female (yin). Positive and negative are just ways to refer to opposite poles. In science you would not think of a negative charge, a negative photograph or the negative pole of a magnet as being worse than its positive counterpart, and it is the same with yinyang. In all these relationships, positive and negative are complementary pairs and each element could not exist or function without the other.

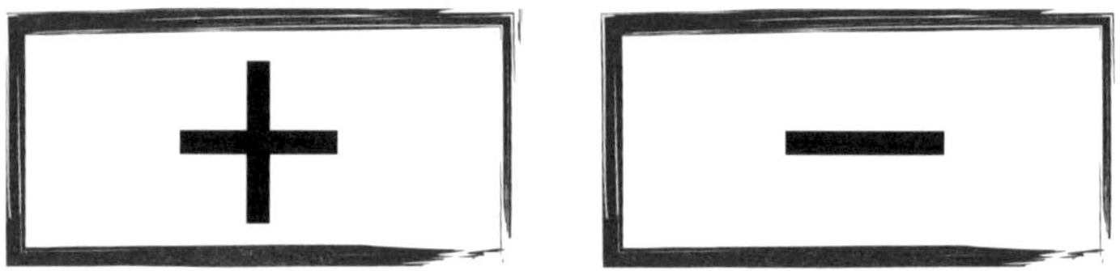

ABOVE: The terms positive and negative refer simply to opposite poles.

☯ Male is yang and yang is positive, female is yin and yin is negative. Positive is not good; negative is not bad. They are just opposites.

STRONG AND WEAK

Yang power is generally more explosive and, therefore, more obvious than yin power, but yin and yang are equally powerful. Yang prevails over yin in the short term only; the sun causes dew to evaporate, fire burns hot and drives out the cold, light removes darkness. However, yang cannot maintain its strength forever; it burns itself out and then yin takes control in more subtle ways until yang bursts into life once more.

Yang overcomes yin and then yin overcomes yang. They take turns to be the stronger, but overall each is as powerful as the other.

INFERIOR AND SUPERIOR

Another dangerous misconception is that yang is superior to yin. Yin and yang are totally equal. Yang may manifest itself in more dramatic ways, but yin is just as influential. For heaven to be healthy it has to have both yin and yang, crops need both sun and rain, and humankind also requires an equal balance of yin and yang. Yinyang represents true equality, and when either yin or yang continually dominates the other, it results in chaos.

Yin and yang are equal, but they have different attributes and perform different roles.

A QUESTION OF CHRONOLOGY

At the beginning of the universe, there was no male and female. There existed just pure yin and yang. It was only billions of years later after humans came into existence that females were categorized as yin and males as yang. So to believe that yin is intrinsically female and yang intrinsically male is to assume that yinyang was invented for humans, which is completely untrue. It is important to remember this.

SENIOR AND JUNIOR

In relationships based on hierarchy, such as that between a teacher and a student, a manager and a worker or an officer and a soldier, the senior person is the yang part while the junior person is the yin. This aspect is completely independent of gender. In terms of seniority, a female manager is yang in relation to a male subordinate, while also being yin in relation to him in terms of gender.

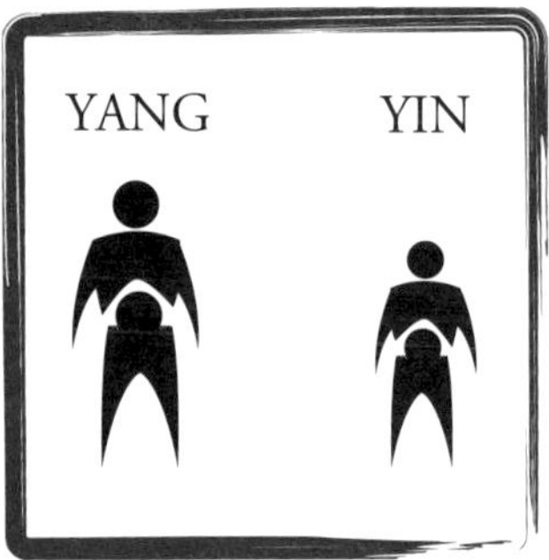

ABOVE: Yang is senior; yin is junior.

Indeed, in any relationship between two people, regardless of gender or hierarchy, one person adopts the yin aspect and the other adopts the yang and together they achieve balance. Sometimes they switch aspects, but the key to a lasting relationship is a balance between yin and yang at any given time. How often do you see people at loggerheads if both of them are too dominant?

Traditionally, yin is associated with the junior party in a relationship and yang with the senior. However, a successful relationship of any kind requires a balance of yin and yang.

FUXI AND MUWA

Yin and yang are equal under the law of heaven. A baking summer drought and a biting winter storm are just as powerful. Chinese mythology portrayed this relationship of equals in male and female terms as the brother and sister Fuxi and Muwa, progenitors of the human race.

In traditional images of the pair, Muwa, the sister, holds a compass of the type used to map the stars, while Fuxi, the brother, holds a set square for measuring land and form. It might seem odd that the yin figure Muwa should hold a symbol of the yang sky and the yang figure Fuxi should hold a symbol of the yin earth. However, the idea is that "sky-father" uses the set square to bind and regulate the earth and its forms, while the "earth-mother" uses the compass to bind and interact with the sky and the formless. This interdependence of yin and yang is also represented in the accompanying illustration of Muwa and Fuxi by the intertwining of the two figures' legs.

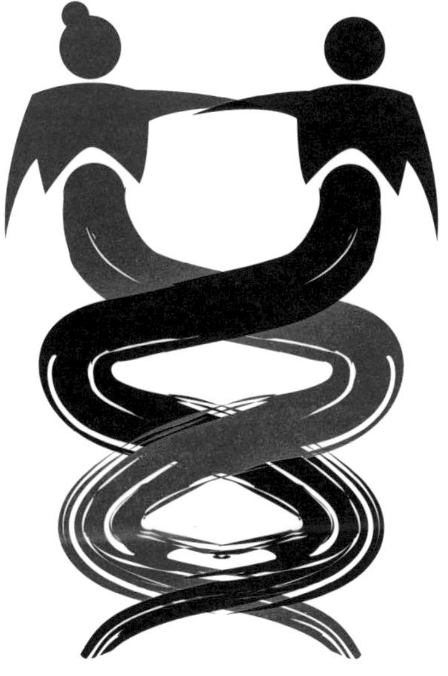

ABOVE: Muwa and Fuxi, the founders of humanity.

☯ **Male and female are intertwined and interdependent, just like yin and yang. Without one, the other does not exist.**

GENDER EQUALITY IN ANCIENT CHINESE SOCIETY

Some Daoist scholars advocated equality between the sexes using analogies such as the so-called "two-hands teaching". They argued that to govern using only men or only women was as restrictive as to use only one hand. A perfect society draws on a proper balance of male and female aspects.

However, many Daoist masters did not share this view and men did become dominant in China. Women and girls suffered in numerous ways, including female infanticide, foot binding and social restrictions. A tradition grew that women ruled inside the home, men ruled outside. Some people fought against this imbalance by pointing out that a male-heavy and male-dominant population went against the laws of yinyang, and that it would cause chaos in the world through an excess of yang energy.

It must also be observed that the inequalities did not run only on gender lines. Imperial China was as much a hierarchy as a patriarchy, with the vast majority of both men and women at the bottom of the pyramid and one man at the top. Yinyang taught equality, but its lessons were not always heard.

Wasting the talents of half of society is like governing with only one hand.

EQUAL BUT DIFFERENT

Yin and yang are truly equal, but have differences in their nature that cause them to prosper in different situations. The sun will not cool you down and the moon will not warm you up, so using the moon for heat and the sun for shade is against the ways of heaven. Likewise, men and women are equal under heaven but, according to yinyang, each person should do what is appropriate to their nature and not force themselves to adopt a role that is against their nature. Some point out that this philosophy can be exploited to confine men and women to certain roles, which risks neglecting the talents of women in traditionally male areas and vice versa.

Although predominantly yang, men contain aspects of yin and, although predominantly yin, women contain aspects of yang. Yinyang theory states that if yang becomes too high in women or yin becomes too high in men, society will become unbalanced and disorderly. According to this theory, men should focus on their yang while maintaining a degree of yin, and vice versa for women. In other words, people should concentrate on the tasks they are most naturally suited to but should also develop abilities that come less easily.

Each person should do what best suits them, while also challenging themselves in areas they find more difficult.

WORKING WITH YINYANG:

Focus on your own yinyang balance, not other people's

Traditional yinyang theory tells us that men are predominantly yang and should develop their yang, while women are yin and should develop their yin, and also that each gender has a smaller part of the opposite element within them. However, gender roles and identities vary between societies and change over time. Gender identity is being questioned and discussed more than ever in the present time. The beauty of yinyang is that, by its very nature, it accommodates fluidity within our existence.

Remember that all people, regardless of gender, are equal under heaven. Let each individual take responsibility for the balance of yinyang within themselves, because if such matters are forced, yinyang will be out of balance and society will start to break down. The way of yinyang is to allow people to live in a natural state in harmony with the landscape without imposing strict social restrictions. Assess your own inner balance of yinyang and let others do the same. Interfering with other people's ways is not the Dao.

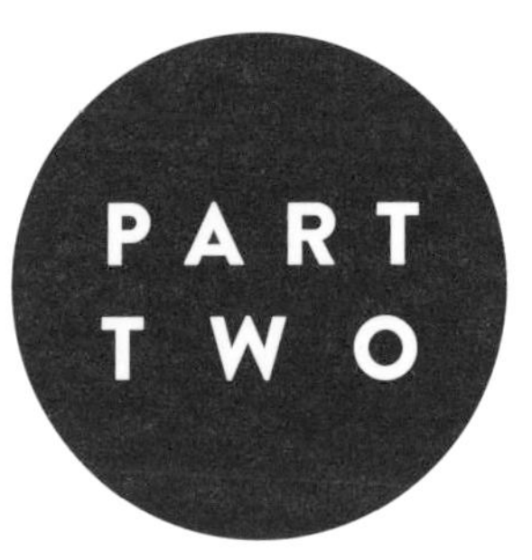

THE HISTORY OF YINYANG

The theory of yinyang developed over many centuries. Simple ideograms for sun and shade on a mountainside date back to the dawn of Chinese writing thousands of years ago. The slow development of a theory based on pairs of natural opposites is known as proto-yinyang. Later, different schools such as Daoism and Confucianism applied complex yinyang systems to government, warfare, medicine, weather forecasting, the study of the heavens, ritual magic and other areas. This part of the book traces the evolution of yinyang into the relatively settled theory that we know today.

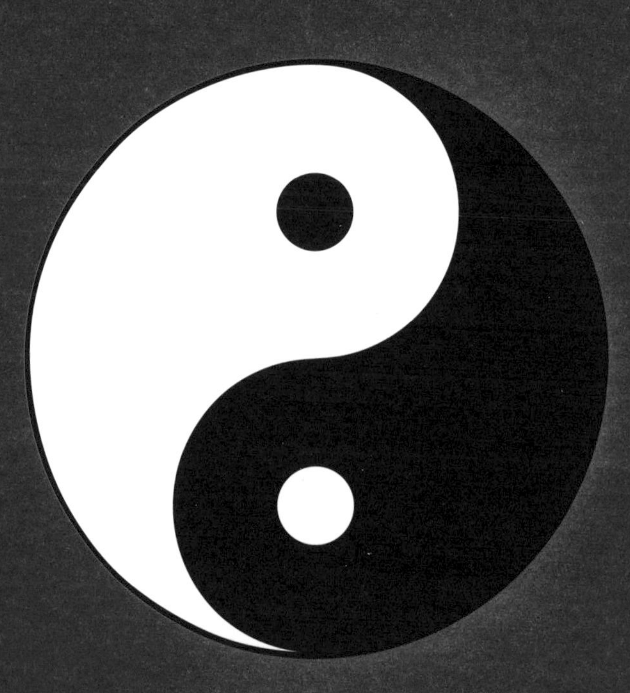

CHAPTER 7

THE BIRTH OF THE UNIVERSE

THE BIRTH OF THE UNIVERSE

Yinyang came into being at the birth of the universe, so to understand the development of yinyang throughout Chinese history we first have to understand how the Chinese thought that the universe was created. There were several competing origin myths dating from the period before China became a single state. Many of them share certain features, most notably a pre-universe that divides into two elements from which all creation follows. In this chapter we will explore the different origin myths in more detail.

THE EGG BEFORE TIME AND SPACE

Before the universe, there was a cosmic egg known as "chaos", and in the middle of this egg was the hero Pangu, who had slept for 800,000 years. When he awoke there was only darkness and so he cracked open the egg in search of light. Pangu started to grow, and for every amount he grew, the sky grew above him and the earth grew below him. The universe continued to grow in this way for another period of 800,000 years.

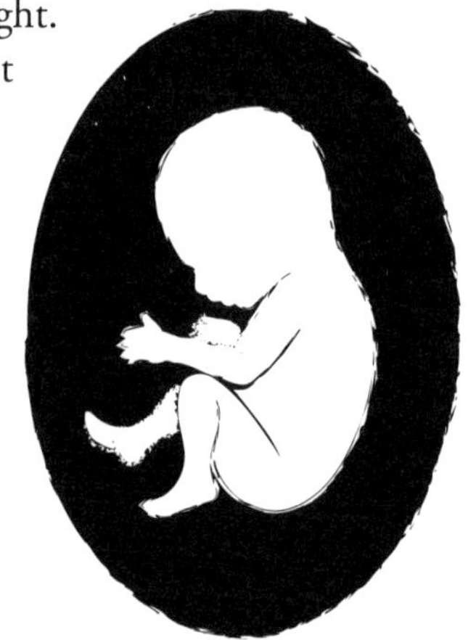

ABOVE: The creator hero Pangu incubating in his cosmic egg.

Eventually Pangu reached his maximum size and died, leaving the sky and the earth complete. His body broke up into "ten thousand things" and created everything on earth and in the sky. His breath became the wind, his voice the thunder; his left eye became the sun, his right eye the moon; his limbs became the four directions and his five major organs became the five sacred mountains of China. Pangu's blood became the waters of the world, while his sweat became the rain, his muscles the soil, his hair the stars, his skin the grass and plants, and his teeth and bones the rocks. Thus was created the world and everything within it. While this origin myth does not mention yinyang, it does follow the other myths in that the universe is born from potential and comes out of chaos or darkness.

The idea of a creator figure hatching from a cosmic egg is also found in Indian, Egyptian and Greek mythology.

THE TEN SUNS

One Chinese legend about the origin of our sun – which is the beginning of our "universe", if not *the* universe – says that originally there were ten suns. They took turns to rise each day, so that while there was only one sun in the sky at any one time they moved around the earth in a ten-day cycle. This is why sometimes the Chinese count periods of ten days, and this corresponds to the 10 Heavenly Stems (see page 156).

One day, all ten suns rose at the same time and burned the ground, destroying life on earth. The emperor of heaven sent forth a great archer to shoot down nine of the suns, leaving only one to rise day after day.

There were once ten suns, before nine of the suns were shot down.

FROM THE ONE TO "TEN THOUSAND THINGS"

The Dao De Jing (see page 93) has a different creation myth, which on the surface appears totally distinct from the others, but people have drawn certain parallels. It says that in the beginning there was "the one". This "one" moved and created "the two", "the two" created "the three" and "the three" created "ten thousand things". The "ten thousand things" were affected by yin and yang and *chi* resonated with harmony in the universe and all burst into life.

The numbers in this myth each have symbolic meaning:

- The one is the Dao.
- The two is yinyang.
- The three is heaven, earth and humans.
- The ten thousand things represent all creation.

All things move from yin (creation) through yang (life) and then return to yin (death). In this version, creation is a never-ending process.

There is a more complex version of the same myth that breaks the emergence of the universe down into more stages. This is called the ultimate manifestation (*taizhao*, 天兆) and can be summarized as follows:

- At the beginning there is nothing but the Dao, which is formless.
- Next comes the generation of time and space.
- Time and space generate *chi*.
- *Chi* begins to move.
- Light *chi* ascends and creates the universe or sky.
- Heavy *chi* congeals and creates matter or earth.
- Yin and yang create the seasons.
- Yang *chi* is the essence of fire and the future sun.
- Yin *chi* is the essence of water and the future moon.
- These aspects of *chi* form the stars and planets, including the earth, sun and moon.

The Dao is always pulsating with yin and yang, and heaven, earth and humans are always being created.

THE CLEAR AND THE TURBID

Within Chinese creation myths you will often hear that clear *chi* ascended and turbid *chi* descended. In the beginning, *chi* changed into heavy yin *chi*, which clumped together and became the ground, and light and radiant yang *chi*, which rose into the sky and became pure air and space.

This process continues to take place every day. Within the space between heaven and earth, clear *chi* rises and heavy *chi* descends. For example, water evaporates and moves up into the sky, as does smoke from a fire. In contrast, rain is dense and falls to the ground, as does ash when the fire cools. Yin and yang *chi* operate unseen to create visible physical phenomena such as fire and rain. The rule is unchanging: light *chi* rises, heavy *chi* descends.

☯ **Yang *chi* radiates outward and upward, while yin *chi* condenses and falls to the ground.**

THE I-CHING VERSION OF CREATION

The famous ancient Chinese work the I-Ching, or Book of Changes, comprises trigrams (images made of three lines) and hexagrams (images made of six lines) and shows a different division in the cosmic order, where each element multiplies to form all of creation.

- The one creates two.
- The two creates four.
- The four creates eight trigrams.
- The eight trigrams create 64 hexagrams.
- The 64 hexagrams create all things in existence.

(See chapter 9 for a more detailed examination of the I-Ching.)

☯ **The trigrams and hexagrams of the I-Ching multiplied to create all things.**

THE MOMENT BEFORE ONE SPLIT INTO TWO

Just before the Great Ultimate split into yin and yang, there was a half-step containing the thought or the possibility of division into two aspects. This is known as *liang yi* (兩儀). The first of the two ideograms that make up this term represents a pair of oxen yoked together. The two oxen are separate but connected and their purpose is singular, but when they are uncoupled from their yoke, they may go in different directions and serve different purposes. This symbolizes yin and yang immediately before the divide.

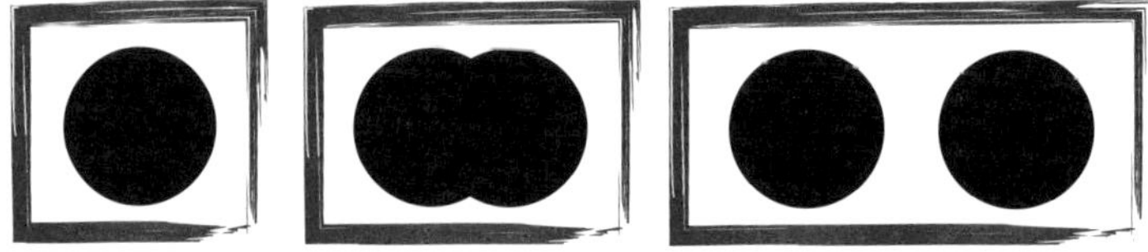

ABOVE: The Great Ultimate *considers* splitting and then divides into yin and yang.

When they were still combined within the one of the Great Ultimate, yin and yang were like two oxen yoked together.

THE ORDER OF THINGS TO COME

One problem that arises in these creation myths is the concept of order and time. We know that the initial division into yin and yang came before the creation of earth and the other planets, the sun, stars and moon, but all things are created from an essence or primordial aspect that predates time and space. The Dao has the essence for creating the universe within it, meaning time and matter are potentials within the pre-universe. The same question occurs in modern scientific theories of how the universe came into being. What was there before time and universal matter?

We know that the splitting of the Great Ultimate into yin and yang is an ongoing and everlasting process. However, what we do not know is how it happened for the first time.

THE WAY IN CHINESE CULTURE

The Way or the Dao appears not only in Daoism but in many other eastern philosophies and religions, including Buddhism and Confucianism, just as the concept of God is found in different western religions. The Way predates all these religions and therefore you should not be puzzled to see it used outside of Daoism.

The Way is a universal concept in Chinese culture. What sets Daoism apart is that it has the Way as its main focus of study.

THE DAO DE JING

Believed to have been written by the sixth-century BC sage Lao Tzu, the Dao De Jing discusses how the universe was created and how humans should exist within the universe. Many scholars see this work as marking the transition from proto-yinyang to the more complex systems of fully fledged yinyang theory. While the text only uses the term yinyang once, in chapter 42, it does so to convey the relatively advanced concept that all things move through yin and yang as states of existence. This moves beyond the primitive idea of yin and yang as the sunshine on a mountain and the shade it creates.

☯ **The Dao De Jing is generally considered the earliest known work of advanced yinyang theory.**

WORKING WITH YINYANG:

Realize that creation is ongoing at all times

Although the details vary, Chinese creation myths tend to describe a pre-universe essence that starts to move and then divides into the manifested parts of creation, a creation that continues to exist and is in a state of constant movement. Look at the world around you and remind yourself that everything is created by the manifestation of yin and yang in movement, made up of a form of binary code which is the physics behind existence. Yin and yang form into countless variations, making the world you live in a pulsating place of divine energy which continues to flow and create time and space. Or alternatively it all came from a giant hero who hatched from a cosmic egg. It is up to you to decide which mythology to enjoy.

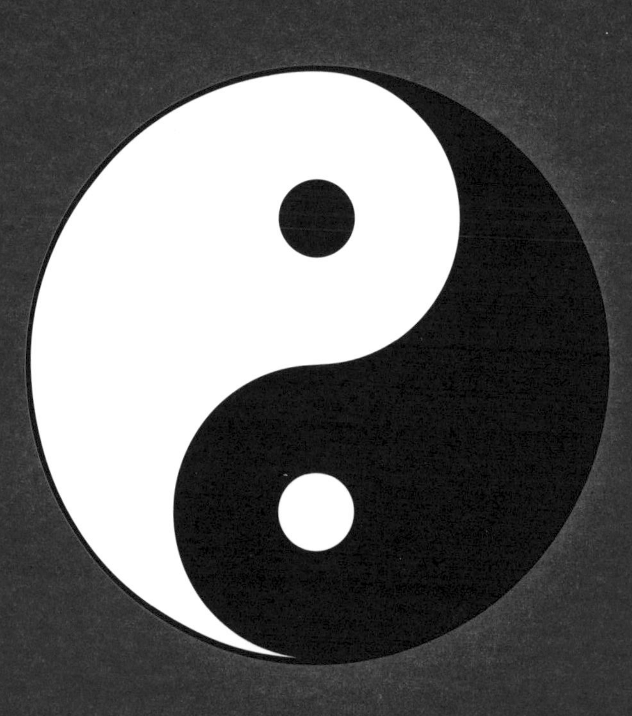

CHAPTER 8

THE SHAPING OF CHINESE SOCIETY

THE SHAPING OF CHINESE SOCIETY

From the first ideograms showing the sun's rays on a hillside to the complex aspects of traditional Chinese medicine, yinyang is a part of China itself. This chapter is an overview of how yinyang has influenced Chinese society and ideas. It is not a chronological analysis of the evolution of the theory but an understanding of the place of yinyang within China and how it helped shape a nation.

THE FIRST SETTLEMENTS

The early Chinese sought places near rivers and open, south-facing land. Yinyang helped identify the positions of these early settlements and then also formed part of their names – for example, in the city names Luo*yang* and Huai*yin*. North is normally associated with yin and south with yang, because the sun is in the south of the sky for all people in the northern hemisphere (see chapter 2). However, for settlements located on the bank of a river, the opposite would be the case. For example, a city on the south bank of a river would have yin in its name. This is because the south bank of a river faces north, making it a shadowy area, which is a yin aspect, while the north bank is open to the sun in the south, making it yang.

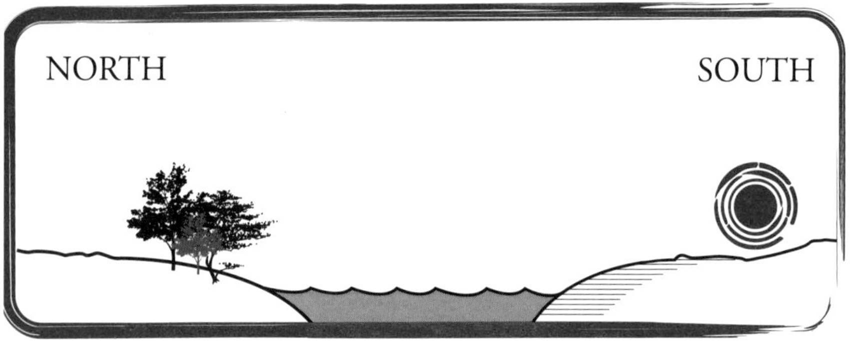

ABOVE: In the northern hemisphere, the south bank of a river is often in shadow because of the position of the sun.

Cities on the shadowy south bank of a river are often named after yin and those on the sunny north bank are often named after yang – this is the opposite of what you would first expect.

THE YELLOW EMPEROR

The mythical Yellow Emperor is generally accepted as an early god who was later portrayed as having ruled China more than 4,000 years ago. His name is often quoted in ancient Chinese sources and he was even revered by the Japanese samurai.

The Yellow Emperor is seen as representing the beginning of the centralization of Chinese culture, the first person to fix down a government and develop Chinese ways. One story tells of how he visited an ancient "master of contemplation" at a place called Hollow Mountain to ask about the secrets of the universe. The master told him that to understand the secrets of the universe he would need to grasp the aspects of heaven and earth, promote the growth of grains, nurture the people and truly understand the rules of yinyang. The emperor was then sent on his way.

After this he abdicated from his throne in search of answers to these points – including the study of yinyang. After a long journey he crawled back to the master at Hollow Mountain on his knees in true submission. The master, who had reached the heights of understanding yang and the depths of understanding yin, went on to teach the Yellow Emperor more secrets, after which he returned to his throne. Endowed with the wisdom of yinyang, the emperor presided over a golden age in China.

Yinyang was at the heart of Chinese government, from the days of the legendary Yellow Emperor more than 4,000 years ago to the end of the imperial era in the early twentieth century.

THE CHINESE PALACE AND GOVERNMENT

In old China, the government was broken up into yin and yang in the following ways:

Emperor (yang)	Empress (yin)

They had their positions within the palace:

Emperor in the south of the palace (yang)	Empress in the north of the palace (yin)

There were six departments:

Office of heaven (yang) overall government and order	Office of earth (yin) education and nourishment
Office of spring (yang) social and religious duties and growth	Office of autumn (yin) justice, punishment and coldness
Office of summer (yang) military and activeness	Office of winter (yin) population, land, agriculture and recuperation

Each office had 60 people working within it; six multiplied by 60 comes to 360, the number of days in the original Chinese year. With all of these sections in place, the Chinese system of government was in alignment with heaven through yinyang.

☯ **The Chinese government was aligned with yinyang so that harmony would reign on earth.**

THE CHINESE DYNASTIES AND THE FIVE PHASES

The Chinese developed a theory that each of their dynasties represented one of the Five Phases (see chapter 16). In Five Phase theory, the different phases or elements – fire, water, wood, metal and earth – interact with each other in what can be seen as either a productive (generative) or destructive (conquering) manner. For example, wood generates fire by acting as fuel, but fire conquers metal by melting it. Here the focus is on conquering, because each dynasty takes over from or conquers the one before it. The following list itemizes the relationships between the first five dynasties.

- The Yellow Emperor, creator of Chinese civilization, was associated with earth.
- The Xia dynasty was associated with wood, which conquers earth.
- The Shang dynasty was associated with metal, which conquers wood.
- The Zhou dynasty was associated with fire, which conquers metal.
- The Qin dynasty was associated with water, which conquers fire.

In this way the ancient Chinese saw the progression of stronger dynasties rising to power. After five dynasties the cycle returned to earth. In reality, the transition from one dynasty to the next was more complex than this system suggests. There were many occasions when numerous factions were vying for the imperial throne. However, from a simplified standpoint, the list above is accurate.

These dynastic changes were predicted by omens from heaven. The Yellow Emperor was foretold by worms and moles coming up from the earth. The colour yellow is the colour of the earth element. The emperor Yu, founder of the Xia dynasty, was foretold by the emergence of evergreens, and so he was of the aspect of wood and his colour was green. Da Yi, the founder of the Shang dynasty, was foretold by metal blades being found in water, so he was of the metal aspect and his colour was white. The rise of King Wen, founder of the Zhou dynasty, was foretold by great fires and red birds, so he was of the fire element and his colour was red. The emperor Qin was of the water element and so his colour was black.

☯ Each Chinese imperial dynasty was associated with one of the Five Phases, which followed on from each other in a cycle. Each phase conquers the previous one just as each dynasty conquered its predecessor.

COLOURS OF THE ELEMENTS

The emperor and his courtiers would dress in the appropriate dynastic colour, as listed above. You will see this in historical dramas set in the various dynasties. You can also often see leaders throughout east Asia wearing yellow, because this is the colour of the earth, which is the centre and foundation for all other elements. The samurai Tokugawa Ieyasu (1543–1616) wore golden yellow armour, possibly because he was the leader of the force and therefore was in a position that reflected the aspect of earth.

Certain Chinese colours cannot easily be translated into other languages. For example, the colour cang *(蒼), which is the colour of newly sprouted spring vegetation, is generally given in English as "blue-green" or something similar but is at times rendered as either "blue" or "green" (in truth, it is close to turquoise). Therefore, be aware that different sources sometimes translate colours in radically different ways.*

RITUALS

Yinyang is central to Chinese ritual culture. An altar can be either yin or yang depending on whether it is facing in a yin or yang direction. Regardless of orientation, the left side of the altar is yang while the right side is yin. In the case of sacrificial rituals, yin animals are chosen for yin rituals and yang ones for yang rituals.

☯ Yinyang influences rituals in various ways, such as the positioning of the altar and the choice of animals to be sacrificed.

WHICH WAY IS WHICH?

When reading directions in old teachings, it is not always clear which way is yang and which way is yin. When there is an instruction to set up in a yin direction, does that mean to be positioned in a yin direction facing yin, or does it mean to be positioned in a yin direction facing yang? Remember, yin and yang directions are relative to the observer, who is central. Consider this: a person setting up on the yin side and facing yin would have their back to the centre and be facing outward toward the right side of the room (right being a direction of yin). Alternatively, if they set up in a yin direction and faced yang, they would have the altar on the right (yin) but face the left part of the room (yang). In truth, it is not always possible to find a satisfactory answer for all problems concerning which way to face when performing a ritual, but always keep these points in mind.

SOCIAL CONTROL

In ancient China, government meant to align human society with the ways of heaven. Humans emit *chi*, which can throw heaven out of balance if too much yin or yang *chi* is emitted. Therefore, if we behave properly, heaven will supply us with everything we need.

The following were practical ways used in old China to govern the population in order to maintain a correct balance of yinyang.

- Use rituals and methods of worship to teach respect.
- Use the principle of yang to instil the ability to adapt and be flexible in thought.
- Use the principle of yin to instil family cohesion and loyalty.
- Use music to teach harmony and relaxation.

If these principles were followed within any community, it was believed there would be peace and prosperity for all.

The whole of society must work to achieve the correct balance of yinyang in order to align with heaven.

THE HORSE AND CHARIOT

The horse was a symbol of military office, and terms with the word horse in them became synonymous with power and duty. The Chinese first encountered the chariot when it was used in battle against them by the Indo-European steppe peoples. They soon adopted it for themselves and it became another statement of power. However, it is when they are put together that the horse and chariot become truly powerful – as a fully realized symbol of the universe.

- The chariot represents the earth.
- The canopy represents heaven.
- The four horses pulling the chariot represent the four seasons.
- The two human drivers represent yin and yang.

The structure of the chariot supports humans just like the earth holds all things up; the canopy protects us like the sky above our heads. The steeds drive us forward just as the four seasons keep propelling us forward through time; and the drivers take turns to steer us to the best place, just as yin and yang take turns to guide us.

Powerful symbols in their own right, the horse and chariot combine to explain the workings of the universe.

THE HUNDRED SCHOOLS

Do not think that ancient China was a place of harmony and culture in which everyone always worked together to maintain a perfect balance of yinyang. It had its share of upheavals, wars, factionalism and changes of dynasty. The concept of yinyang goes back into prehistoric times, but as Chinese civilization grew, diverse ideas from all parts of the land competed for supremacy. This process, which took place from the sixth to the third century BC, is known as the Hundred Schools of Thought. As well as scholars from the yinyang school, there were Confucianists, Legalists, Daoists, Mohists, Logicians and so on, all of whom came together to argue over the correct way to govern China. Within each school there were multiple factions, so there was certainly no end of debate. However, yinyang persisted as a fundamental idea for the way the universe worked.

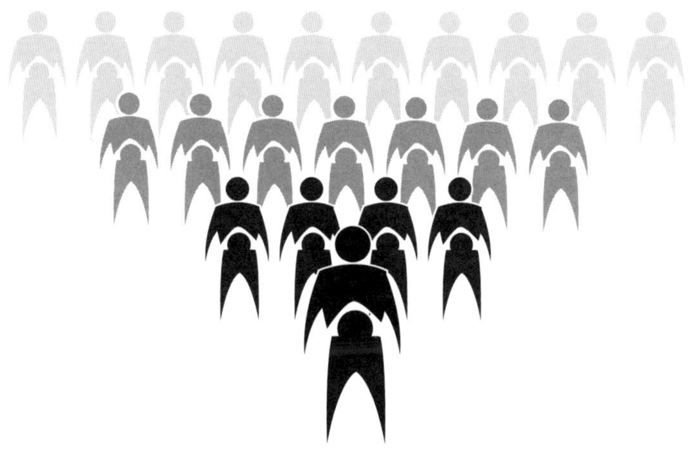

ABOVE: Each school of thought broke down into various factions.

Yinyang was just one of many schools of thought in ancient China. However, while most of the schools have fallen away, including the yinyang school, their ideas have survived into the modern age.

THE SCHOOL OF YINYANG

The school of yinyang was called *yinyangjia* (陰陽家), "the house of yinyang". In some books you will see its adherents referred to as "the Naturalists", because they dealt with nature, the origin of the earth and heavens and the continuous process of creation.

The yinyang school is believed to have evolved from within Confucianism, one of the major schools of thought in ancient China. Also known as *rujia*, Confucianism was the realm of the gentleman (士), people from a high social class who had the time to engage in such studies. It included a group of people known as *fangshi* (方士), "gentlemen of skills and techniques", who adopted old folk customs (they would all have been men in this time). It was to this subgroup that the term yinyang school was loosely applied. One particular *fangshi* gentleman known as Tsou Yen (c.305–240 BC) is mentioned in the Records of the Great Historian (145–86 BC) as having been a prominent figure in the yinyang school, but everything he wrote is now lost.

Although most of the school's teachings have not survived, the basic elements can be pieced together from various documents to form an understanding of yinyang theory. However, without knowing how much of the whole picture of yinyang has been lost, it is hard to say just how full our understanding is.

The actual school might have died out, but the concept of yinyang continued to influence many areas of Chinese life. The following list of arts within the yinyang curriculum has been reconstructed from the writings of other schools about yinyang.

- Observing the heavens
- Calendar calculation
- Good fortune
- Prohibitions
- Taboos
- Rituals
- Music
- Numerology
- Ghosts and spirit lore
- Dream lore
- Physiognomy
- Alchemy
- Sex, magic and rituals
- The four seasons
- The Five Phases
- The eight positions
- The 12 measures
- The 24 restrictions

From what we know about the school of yinyang it appears to have been highly esoteric, with interests ranging from music to ghost lore.

THE CHINESE CALENDAR

Today in the West we use the Gregorian calendar, which keeps the year in alignment with the solstice and the equinox and observation of the sun and earth. The Chinese use a lunisolar calendar, originally called the yinyang calendar. It follows the cycles of the moon and sun and needs to be adjusted annually to maintain alignment. This is why Chinese New Year changes date each year. In Chinese writing the ideogram for "day" (日) also means "sun" because the sun appears each day and the ideogram for "month" (月) also means "moon" because each month lasts 28 days, the length of a lunar cycle. Measuring months by the cycle of the moon meant that some years had 12 months and others had 13; these were known as lesser and greater years.

☯ **The dates of the Chinese calendar are not the same as those of the western calendar. Problems can arise when attempting to mix the two.**

CHINESE COINS

Previously we encountered the idea that the earth (yin) is represented as a square because of the angles of the earth, while the sky (yang) is represented as a circle because the sky is a dome above our heads. This symbolism is replicated within Chinese coins, which are sometimes known as square-hole coins. The coin itself is round and has a square hole in the centre; this represents the globe of the sky (yang) surrounding the square earth (yin). (There is also a practical reason for Chinese coins to have a hole in the middle, which is so that they could be strung together for ease of handling. However, that does not take away from their symbolic meaning.)

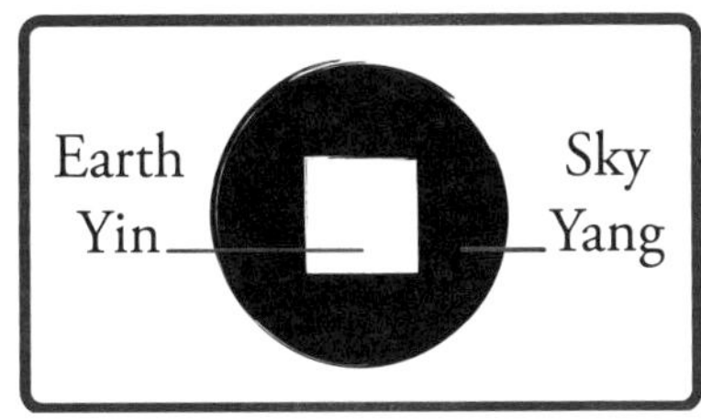

ABOVE: A Chinese square-hole coin representing the dome of the sky and the angles of the earth.

What makes this representation particularly interesting is that the sky, which is formless in real life, is represented by the solid metal of the coin; while the earth, which is solid in real life, is represented by the void in the middle. This is thought to be connected to the principle of *you-wu*, or "presence and absence". As well as symbolizing the interaction of yin and yang, the coin represents the presence of things that exist and the absence of things that have the potential to exist in the future.

With its circular form surrounding a square hole, a Chinese coin is the physical embodiment of heaven encircling earth.

THE HUMAN BODY AS HEAVEN AND EARTH

Like the Chinese coin, the human body is seen as symbolizing earth and heaven, yin and yang. The head at the top is round like the globe of the sky and it points upward to heaven. The point at the crown of the head specifically represents the North Star, Polaris. The feet at the bottom point downward and when put together make a square shape, representing the angles of the earth. Urine, the water of the body, is salty and moves downward, just like the seas upon the surface of the earth.

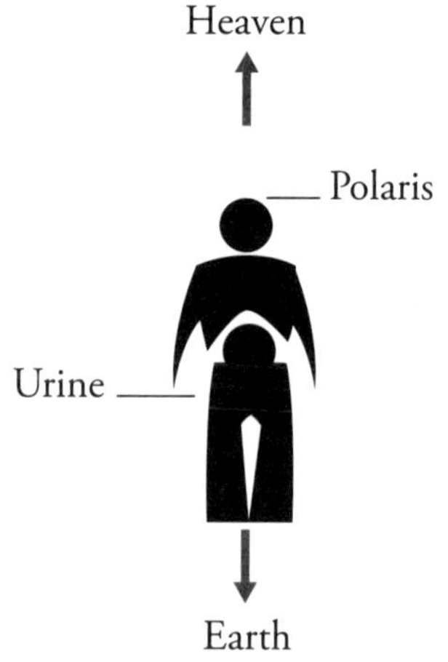

ABOVE: The circle (head) and square (feet) of the human body, symbolizing heaven and earth.

In this way, the human body was seen as being aligned in the correct manner, with heaven above and earth below. The people of the ancient East took this vertical stance as evidence of human superiority over other animals, which tend to have a horizontal alignment.

With its round head at the top like the sky above and its feet at the bottom representing the angles of the earth below, the human body is in a proper relationship with the universe.

THE SQUARE DANCE

Priests in the Daoist tradition perform a ritual dance to celebrate the moment when order came from chaos and yin and yang came into harmony. This dance is done in a square that has nine squares within it, typical of the "magic square" seen in other ritual practices.

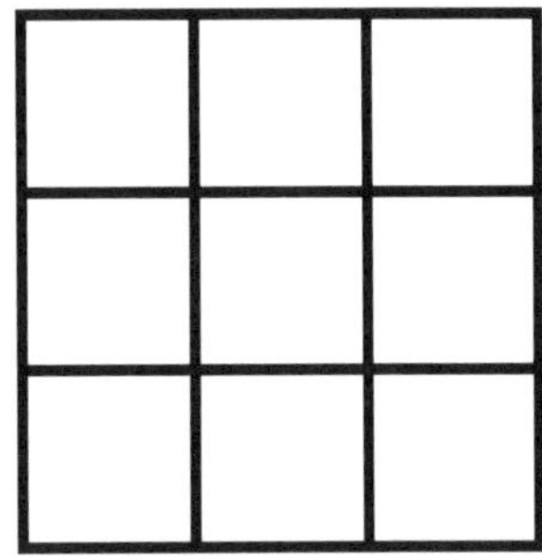

ABOVE: The magical nine square

The nine square represents both yin and yang – yin because it is a square, the shape of the earth, and yang because nine is the highest yang number. The priest dances within each square, building up the full power of yinyang. Note that this dance takes place only once every 60 years, at the culmination of the 60-year cycle on which the Chinese calendar is based.

The ritual square dance celebrates the moment when yinyang came into being.

THE YINYANG SYMBOL

Also known as the *taiji*, the world-famous yinyang symbol is a much later idea than yinyang itself, but has come to be emblematic of the dynamic union of yin and yang.

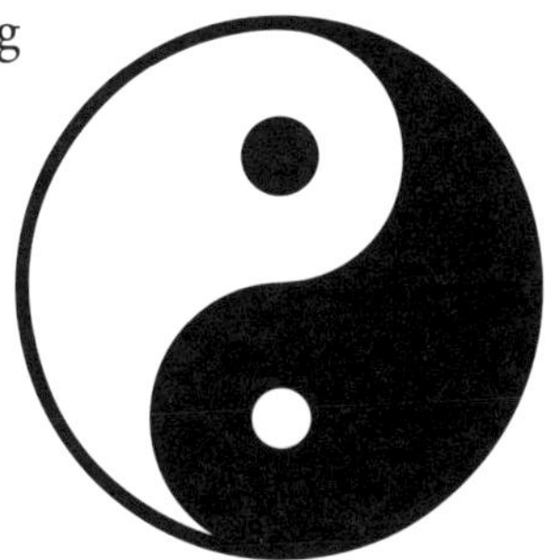

ABOVE: The yinyang *taiji*.

Versions of the *taiji* started to appear in Daoist iconography by the year 1000. It manages to capture in a static image the swirling movement of yin and yang as they are born, grow, recede, die and give way to their opposite. The white, which is yang, is on the left and rises up to the top just like the yang sun; while the black, which is yin, is on the right and represents the sun setting in the west. Note that the swirling should be visualized as a clockwise movement. This perpetual rise and fall of the two elements is what keeps the world moving.

The two small dots represent the birth of the new element. Yin grows out of yang and yang grows out of yin in a never-ending cycle. Destruction carries generation within it and life has to have death to continue.

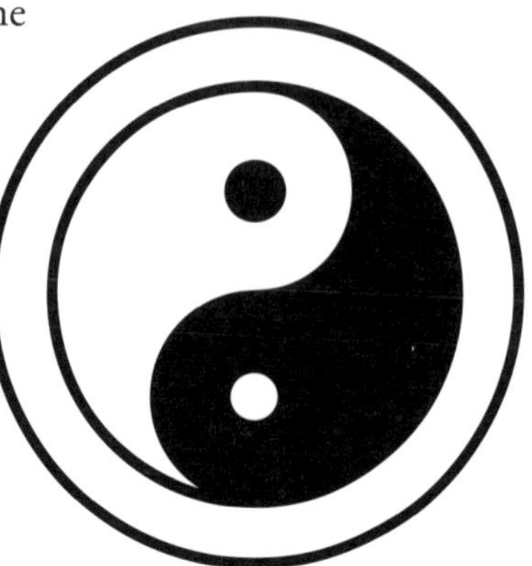

ABOVE: Sometimes the symbol has a circle around it to represent the Great Ultimate and underline the pivotal role of yinyang in the creation of the universe.

The *taiji* has been likened to two fish swimming together (it is sometimes known as the fish symbol) or two rushing rivers intertwining or the sun and moon circling each other in the heavens.

☯ **The swirling yinyang symbol known as the *taiji* perfectly conveys the perpetual movement from yin to yang and yang to yin.**

A ROMAN CONNECTION?

There is a theory that the Chinese obtained this symbol from the Romans, as a similar symbol in black and gold with two red dots appears in the late Roman document the Notitia Dignitatum.

ALTERNATIVE YINYANG SYMBOLS

Before the *taiji* came to prominence, other symbols and diagrams including the *taijitu* and *wujitu* were used to represent the concept of yinyang and the universe.

THE *TAIJITU* – A MAP OF THE UNIVERSE

The *taijitu* diagram (top right) shows how everything starts in the Great Ultimate or the void at the top and moves down into yinyang. This generates the Five Phases and from them come the men and women of the human race. This is an illustration of how the universe was born and the place of yinyang within it.

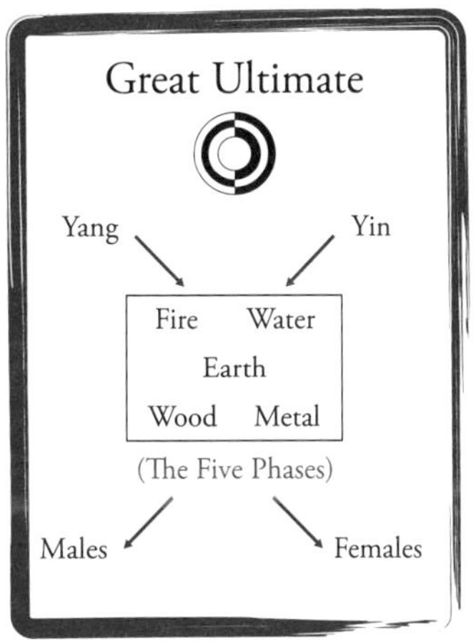

THE *WUJITU* – A WAY BACK TO THE DIVINE

The *wujitu* diagram (bottom right) looks similar to the *taijitu*, but it is read the opposite way – that is to say, from bottom to top. It shows how a human can return to the Great Ultimate through internal alchemy. It starts at the gate at the bottom, where one has to understand self-perfection, then moves to self-cultivation to acquire divinity. Through the connection between the Five Phases and *chi* with an understanding of internal yinyang, a person can arrive at a state of purity and emptiness. Once this state is reached, only then upon death will they return to the Great Ultimate or the essence of the universe.

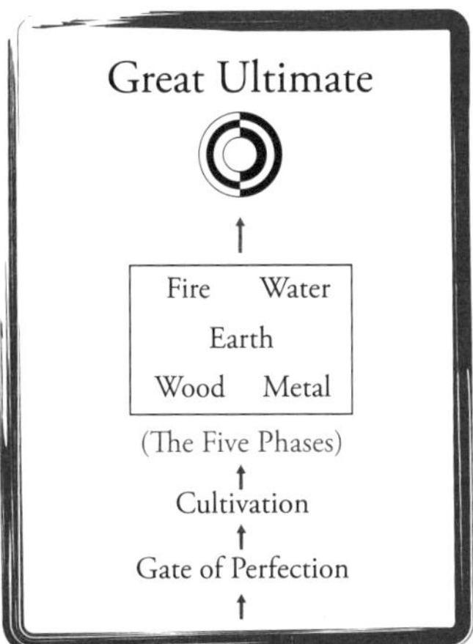

ABOVE: The *taijitu* (top) is read from top to bottom, while the *wujitu* (bottom) is read from bottom to top.

The *taijitu* and *wujitu* remind us that the universe is an engine of creation and destruction, which pulsates with energy that gives form but also dissolves and returns to the place of origin.

GOOD AND EVIL

Some scholars have suggested a connection between the Middle Eastern religion of Zoroastrianism and yinyang theory. Zoroastrianism is centred around the concept of two forces working against each other, the forces of light and the forces of dark; good versus evil. This sounds similar to yinyang on the surface, but there is an important difference: yinyang is about the movement of change between two opposites, neither of which is good or bad. Although both revolve around duality, there is a distinct contrast between the western concept of good versus evil, God versus the Devil, and the eastern idea of two complementary elements moving in and out of phases. Buddhism goes one step further, maintaining that the goal of existence is to move beyond duality, to extinguish the part that is consciousness and transcend the cycles of life and death and the known universe.

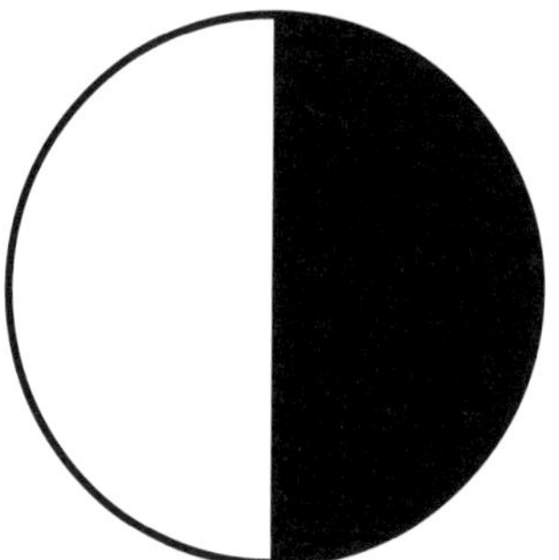

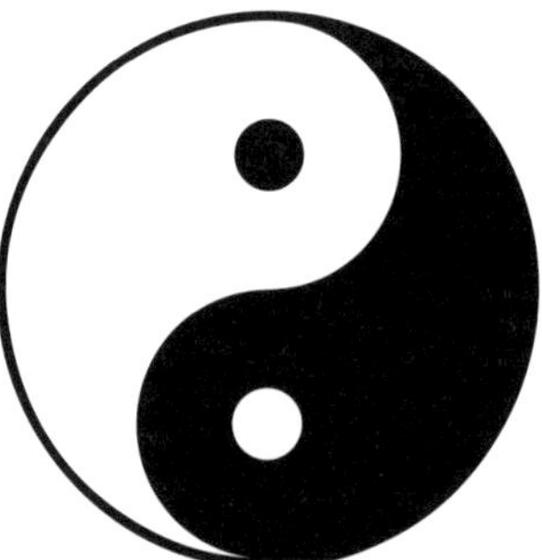

ABOVE: The western idea of good facing off against evil (left) differs from the yinyang concept of two opposite forces moving in unison to create the world (right).

THE UNIVERSE IN DOTS

The scholars of *tushu*, the "school of diagrams and writings", sought to understand the universe through visual representations. They produced images called *tu* (圖), meaning "diagrams", which used black and white dots to represent yinyang and sometimes incorporated animals such as horses and tortoises. These *tu* diagrams have a wide history and convey many complex systems of thought. The drawings can represent the ownership of knowledge or were sometimes used as a focus for meditation and contemplation.

The dots themselves hold multiple meanings: their colour, the lines that connect them, their position, whether they are odd or even in number, and the total number – all have significance. For example, some diagrams have 55 dots, which in some systems is the number that represents heaven, whereas other diagrams have 45, the number of earth. Furthermore, the dots may be arranged in a circle to represent heaven or a square to represent earth.

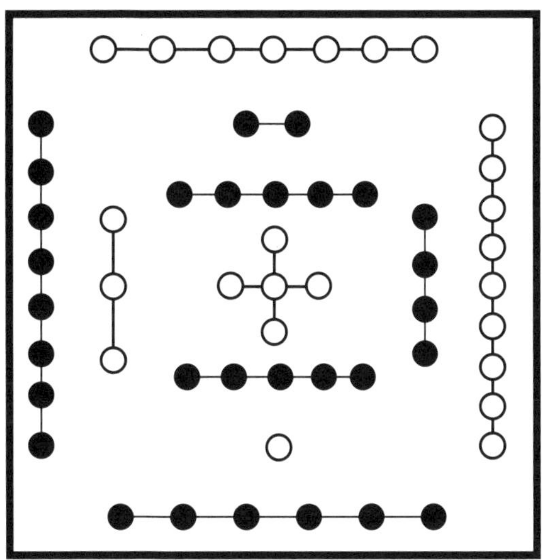

ABOVE: An example of a *tu* diagram.

☯ *Tu* diagrams use arrangements of dots to represent the universe.

THE DANGER OF MIXING SYSTEMS

One big problem that we have today when we look back at ancient China is understanding how everything fits together. Is this writer a Daoist? Are they a Confucianist? Or are they a spirit-talker? It is hard to know where the boundaries lie. While the different ideologies of the various schools clashed, sometimes violently, their teachings do seep into one another and share many common themes. For example, the Way is found in Daoism, Buddhism and even Confucianism.

Things become even more complicated when you start to look at concepts that have no clear label to describe them. Often folklore, magic and shamanism are thrown in with Daoism, even if they have no connection to it at all. Likewise, in Japan, Shinto is often made to absorb all kinds of native folklore and ritual.

The result is a mass of wisdom and knowledge falling under countless labels, all of which is mixed together in the swirl of time and lost records. Teachings that resemble each other in some ways contradict each other in others. Therefore, never be disheartened if you do not fully understand a particular concept, because no one really understands it all. Take peace in the thought that these teachings of the Buddha, the Daoist sages, Confucius and others have enriched the lives of people across the ages and throughout Asia – as they now have the potential to enrich your life.

☯ The three great religions of China – Buddhism, Daoism and Confucianism – all had their place in Chinese society and shaped ancient Chinese wisdom.

WORKING WITH YINYANG:

Study yinyang in all its aspects

For much of its history yinyang was a simple, universal idea – the basis for the Chinese world view. It was only later that it was codified and systemized, with many extra layers of complexity added. Understand that the fundamental aspects of yinyang are rooted in the landscape and the cycles of nature, but also that yinyang as a concept was developed by the elite and given sophistication beyond local folk practices. To follow the way of yinyang you have to engage with it on all levels, seeing it in the landscape and in the theory of creation, studying it in intricate systems of thought, in symbolic representations such as coins and diagrams, and as a way of living that appears throughout society. When pursuing these different manifestations of yinyang, be careful not to detach too much from its natural flow.

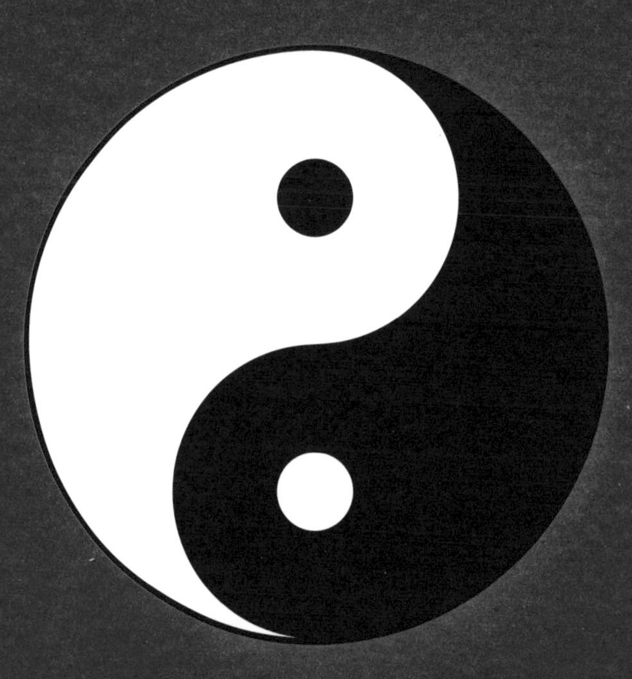

CHAPTER 9

THE I-CHING

THE I-CHING

Almost everyone has heard of the I-Ching. Even if you cannot recall where you have encountered it, as you read on you will start to recognize symbols from it and know that somehow it has entered your life at least once. To call the I-Ching a book is problematic, because it is actually a collection of 64 symbols with attached commentary. It does not read like a book at all, but instead appears complex to the point of being indecipherable. This chapter will attempt to deconstruct the whole mysterious volume and explain its place in history, its purpose and, of course, its connection to yinyang.

WHAT IS THE I-CHING?

The I-Ching (易經) is one of the oldest books in the world, although it took many centuries to evolve into its finished state. Believed to have originated in around 1100 BC, it had developed into a more coherent text by 300 BC but the classic version we know today was not finalized until 1715 AD, in what is now known as the Palace Edition.

Essentially, it consists of a list of hexagrams (a symbol of six lines). Each hexagram is made up of two trigrams (a symbol of three lines). There are eight trigrams, which can be combined in 64 different ways to make the 64 hexagrams of the I-Ching.

The main purpose of the book is to enable the user to stay one step ahead by understanding the changes that are about to occur in a given situation and by making correct decisions to take account of those changes. Originally the I-Ching was about predicting the changes in an external situation. However, later, after it had passed through many factions and commentators, the book also came to give guidance on inner changes.

Normally, the title is translated as the "Book of Changes". However, the first ideogram in the title (易) has four original meanings: "simplicity", "changing", "divination" and "consistency", so "the book of easy and consistent changes through divination" would be a fuller translation.

☯ The I-Ching is a divination tool to help us anticipate changes and take the correct action.

HOW TO SAY IT

The correct pronunciation of the I-Ching is "ee-Ching" or "yee-Ching", not "eye-Ching".

HOW DOES THE I-CHING WORK?

A person wanting to know what changes they should make in their life should first formulate a question they want help answering and then cast a fortune. This is done by throwing a set of three coins six times or casting sticks to build a hexagram. This hexagram will either be considered as static, meaning it does not change and it is the only hexagram you will need to interpret in the divination, or the hexagram will have one or more transforming lines, which will give rise to an additional hexagram to use in the divination. More will be explained on this later.

☯ A person using the I-Ching builds their personal reading by throwing coins or casting sticks.

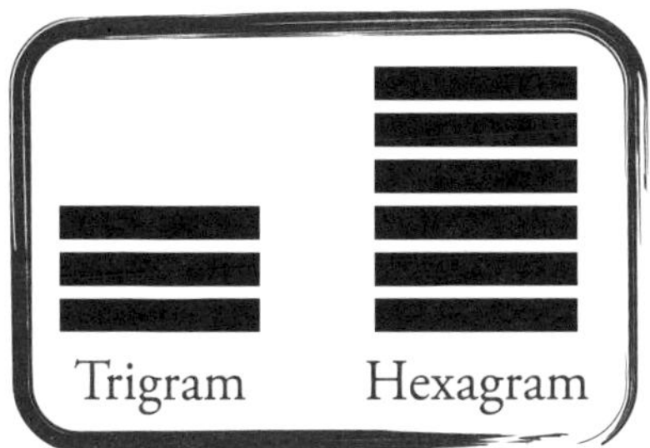

ABOVE: A trigram (left) is a combination of three lines; a hexagram (right) combines two trigrams to make six lines.

A SHORT HISTORY OF LINE DIVINATION

The migratory clans of prehistoric China had so-called "spirit-talkers", who were believed to be able to communicate with the dead and act as a bridge to the divine otherworld. People would go to the spirit-talker with questions they wanted the spirits behind the veil of life to answer. The spirit-talker would take the shoulder bones of sacrificial animals to a fire and, in a state of meditation or trance, would ask the question and apply heat and fire to the bones with a hot brand or stick. This would cause the bone to crack, producing lines that were interpreted for an answer.

From shoulder bones they progressed to tortoise shells, which produced more complex systems of lines. The tortoise as an animal for divination was not picked at random; the upper part of the shell represents the dome of heaven, which is above the flat surface of the earth, represented by the flat underside of the shell. The inside of the tortoise shell represents the space in which creation lives between heaven and earth. This makes the tortoise a perfect symbolic representation of the three realms of heaven, earth and humans.

The cracks appeared as burn circles, crack clusters, T-shapes, shallow arrows, horizontal crosses, split-vertical lines and an X variant. Some of these lines developed into the ideograms used by the Chinese to represent numbers, such as the ones for "eight" (八) and "nine" (九). Eventually, the various cracks in these bones and shells were simplified into two types of line: the solid yang line and the split yin line. The eight trigrams and 64 hexagrams of the I-Ching are all made up of different combinations of these two lines. At a certain point, the lines were given numerical values and this became an important part of I-Ching divination.

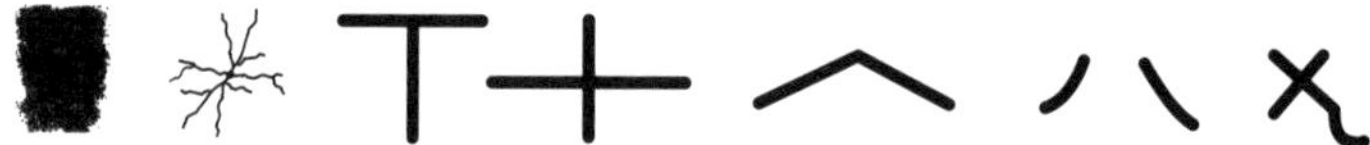

ABOVE: The various types of line found in old divination practice.

☯ The solid yang lines and split yin lines that make up the hexagrams of the I-Ching derive from burn marks made on tortoise shells and the shoulder bones of sacrificial animals.

THE LEGEND OF THE I-CHING

As we have seen, the I-Ching developed gradually over centuries. Various dynasties, such as the Han and the Song, and schools of thought, such as the Buddhists and Neo-Confucianists, made changes and additions until eventually the work became standardized in 1715.

However, there is another, legendary version of how the I-Ching originated. In this version, which can be seen as a kind of creation myth, the book was the work of four individual people who contributed to it in the following stages:

1. The legendary Fuxi, who founded humanity with his sister, Muwa, recorded the eight trigrams.
2. The Count of the West developed the 64 hexagrams from the eight trigrams.
3. King Wen interpreted the hexagrams and organized them into the classic order that we know today.
4. Confucius studied the text and wrote commentaries on it. The I-Ching became one of the "Five Classics" of Confucianism.

When you come across this "history", know that, while it may contain elements of truth, it is not the correct story.

☯ The legend of the I-Ching, that it was created in four stages by Fuxi, the Count of the West, King Wen and Confucius, should be treated with caution.

THE MAWANGDUI MANUSCRIPT

In 1973 a collection of ancient Chinese manuscripts written on silk was discovered at Mawangdui in Hunan. Among the works was an alternative version of the I-Ching. Dated to 168 BC, making it one of the earliest known examples of the text, it arranged the hexagrams in a different order from the classic version and also gave different names to 35 of the 64 hexagrams.

THE CONTENTS OF THE I-CHING

The I-Ching contains a combination of divination and philosophy. The original divination section, which consists of the 64 hexagrams, is accompanied by a commentary called the Ten Wings, which was added later and is broken into three areas:

- an overall understanding of the system
- commentary on each of the 64 hexagrams
- instructions for divination

The book is an extremely complex text that requires years of study to understand it fully. However, it is accessible on many levels and you should not be discouraged from engaging with it. Just be aware that there are pitfalls to avoid and that it is an index to be consulted not a work to be read from start to finish like a normal book.

☯ **The I-Ching is a complex text to be treated with respect.**

PROBLEMS OF TRANSLATION

The art of translating the ideas and intentions of an author from one culture and language to another is difficult enough. With the I-Ching there is the additional problem of time: most of the text is ancient and there is great debate over the original meanings of some of the ideograms, meanings which have changed throughout the expansive history of China. For example, a term that originally meant "to gather" later became used to refer to "military troops". Therefore, to gain the fullest possible understanding of the text you would need to study multiple translations, footnotes and commentaries – a lifelong task indeed.

THE LINES OF YIN AND YANG

The 64 hexagrams of the I-Ching each comprise a different combination of six solid and broken lines. The solid lines are yang and the broken lines are yin. The following is an overview of the lines and their evolution and classification.

THE EARLIER YIN AND YANG LINES BEFORE STANDARDIZATION

As we have seen, the early version of the I-Ching found at Mawangdui had different names for some hexagrams and a different order from the classic Palace Edition of 1715. Each line has a numerical value; the ones in the Mawangdui manuscript used a form of numbering that predated the standardized Chinese system.

THE STANDARD YIN AND YANG LINES

Later in Chinese history the lines became standardized into the formations that are well known today. These consist of either a solid line (yang) or a broken line (yin).

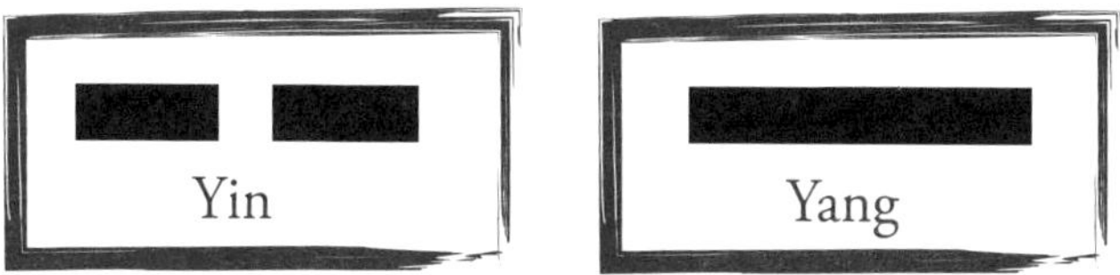

ABOVE: A yin line is made up of two halves with a gap between the two sections; a yang line is a single solid line.

OLD AND YOUNG LINES

The lines are subdivided into old and young, giving four types of line in total: old yang, young yang, old yin and young yin. (Some texts use the terms "greater" instead of "old" and "lesser" instead of "young".) The following section will explain how you get each type of line. For now, what you need to know is that young lines are fixed, whereas old lines transform. This means that if you cast a hexagram made up entirely of young lines, your divination will be based only on that hexagram. However, any old lines in your hexagram will change (yin to yang or yang to yin) to create an extra hexagram that you will need to interpret in addition to your original hexagram. Each hexagram has its own name and interpretation.

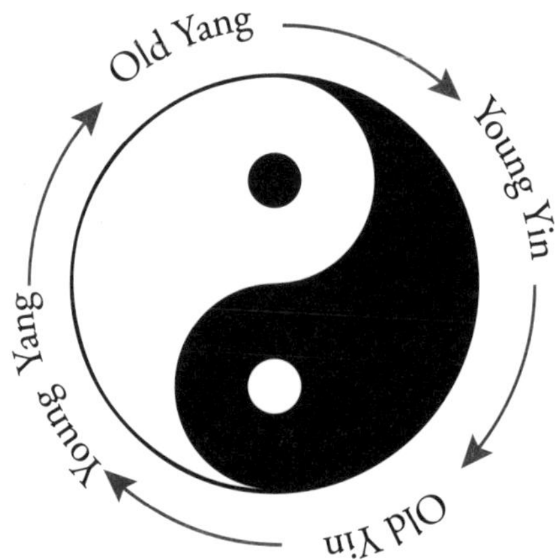

ABOVE: Old yang transforms into young yin and old yin transforms into young yang.

Why do young lines stay the same and old lines transform? Think of the difference between the young yang energy of the rising sun, when yang is set to remain in prominence for the rest of the day, and the old yang energy of the setting sun, when yang is soon to change to yin. Likewise, the young yin energy at nightfall compared with the old yin energy at daybreak.

Be careful, if you do not get this right you will read from the wrong hexagram.

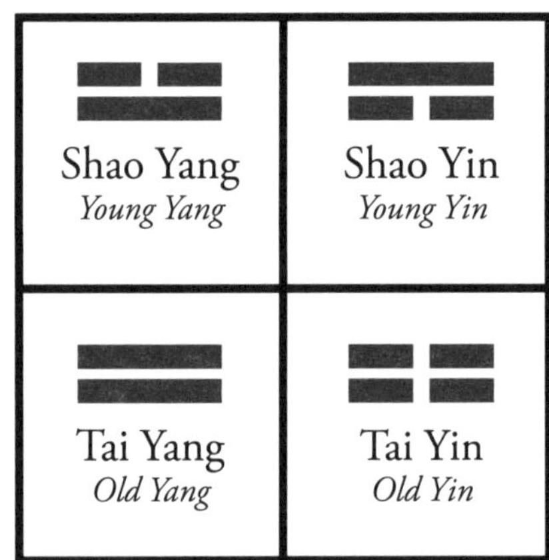

ABOVE: Young and old yin and yang lines and their traditional Chinese names.

The 64 hexagrams are constructed from a combination of solid yang lines and broken yin lines. Yin and yang lines can be either young or old. Young lines are fixed; old lines transform.

CASTING A HEXAGRAM

To use the I-Ching you need to cast a hexagram from which you can get your personal reading. Using the three-coin method, the process is relatively straightforward. There are one or two stumbling blocks to look out for, but overall it is the interpretation of the hexagram that requires more care.

The most important thing to understand about coin divination is that it is a way to get either a yin or yang result. If you look online you will find many ways to do this, each of which claims to be the "correct" system. One of the most common involves giving numerical values to each side of the coins (typically, two for heads and three for tails) and then adding up the three values from each toss to give a total that equates to either a yin or yang line.

Here we will put the numerical system to one side and go back to the basics of yin and yang. A coin has a front (heads) and a back (tails); the front is considered yang and the back is considered yin. When you cast using the three-coin method you can only ever end up with four variations:

- Three yang sides
- Three yin sides
- Two yang sides and one yin side
- Two yin sides and one yang side

There are no results other than these.

Each cast of the three coins will build a single line of your hexagram, starting with the bottom line and working up. After casting six times you will have completed your hexagram and will now have to consider if it is a transforming hexagram or a static one. This is where the first major issue arises, as there are multiple, conflicting versions of this process. Two of the most common are given below.

YIN YIN YIN =
YIN YIN YANG =
YANG YANG YIN =
YANG YANG YANG =

ABOVE: Version one. Note that in both versions red lines transform into their opposite; black lines stay as they are.

Here a throw of three yin sides (tails) represents a transforming yin line, and a throw of three yang sides (heads) represents a transforming yang line. These lines transform into their opposite: yin to yang and yang to yin. However, a throw of two yin sides and one yang side represents a static yang line; and two yang sides and one yin side gives a static yin line. The reasoning behind this counter-intuitive system is not known.

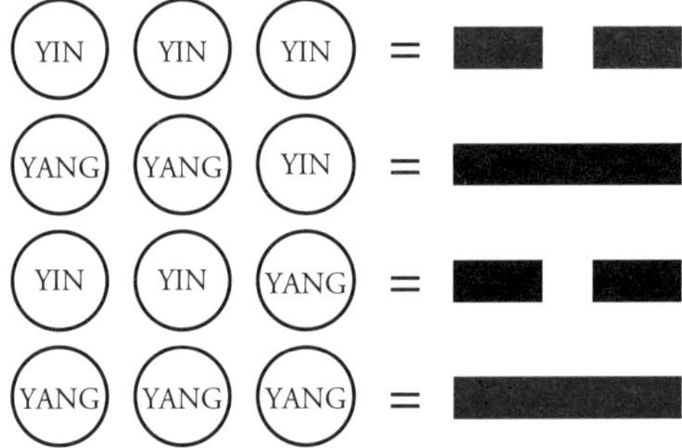

ABOVE: Version two. The difference here is that a predominantly yin throw gives a static yin line and a predominantly yang throw gives a static yang line.

In the second version, all-yin or all-yang throws are treated in the same way as in the first version. However, notice that the mixed pair of throws shown in the middle are the other way round compared to the first version. A throw of two yang sides and one yin creates a static yang line, whereas a throw of two yin sides and one yang creates a static yin line.

How can it be possible that there are two or even more versions? Surely there should be only one system? Do not let such contradictions discourage you from using the I-Ching. Your coin tossing is a question to the Dao or to the spirits beyond the veil of the material world. As long as you are consistent in your approach there will be no problem. The Dao is outside of time and space; it saw the way your coins landed before you even decided to do a reading. Therefore, rest assured that as long as you are clear which version you are using and you make your intent firm in your mind, the Dao will do the rest. All you have to worry about now is which lines transform.

DEALING WITH TRANSFORMING LINES

If you get any "old" lines in your fortune (the red lines in the images attached) when you cast your hexagram, you will end up with two hexagrams to use: the original one and the transformed hexagram. Both of these play a role in the I-Ching fortune. The following example shows how old yin and old yang lines in the primary hexagram change into young yang and young yin lines respectively in the transforming hexagram.

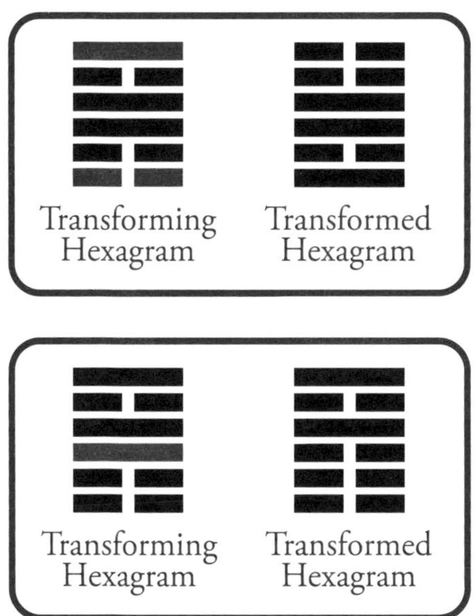

ABOVE: The old lines in the primary hexagram (shown in red) become their opposite in the second, transforming hexagram.

Simply write out both hexagrams, the primary one and then the new, transforming one. And continue on to your reading.

Primary hexagrams are built from the bottom line up. Any old lines transform into their opposite, giving rise to a second hexagram to be interpreted.

YINYANG AS BINARY CODE

The lines of yin and yang can be converted into binary code: a yin line appears as a zero and a yang line as a one. Each trigram and hexagram – and, technically, the whole of existence – can be represented as a string of ones and zeroes.

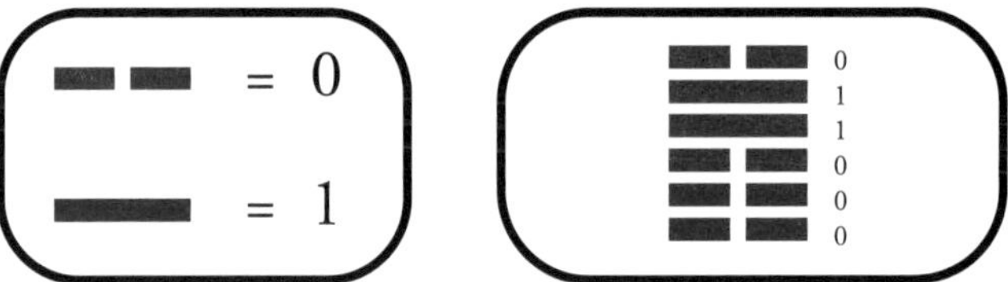

ABOVE: Converting yin and yang lines into binary code.

THE EIGHT TRIGRAMS

There are only eight different ways of combining yin and yang lines in sets of three. These permutations are known as the eight trigrams and each has a meaning deriving from an observable natural phenomenon.

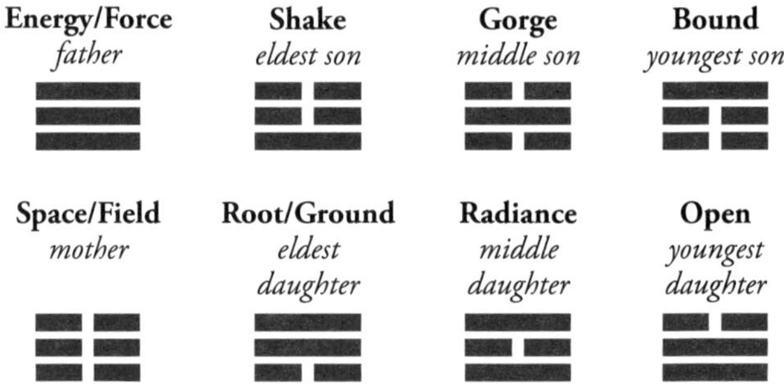

ABOVE: The basic associations for each of the trigrams.

However, take note that there are variations in the way these meanings have been translated and there may be additional connotations ascribed to each trigram. The table below contains information about each trigram based on the English translation by Daoist master Alfred Huang (born 1921).

Trigram	Name	Symbol	Action	Family Order
☰	*Qian*	Heaven	Persisting	Father
☷	*Kun*	Earth	Yielding	Mother
☳	*Zhen*	Thunder	Stirring-up	Eldest Son
☵	*Kan*	Water	Venturing / Falling	Middle Son
☶	*Gen*	Mountain	Stopping	Youngest Son
☴	*Xun*	Wood / Wind	Entering	Eldest Daughter
☲	*Li*	Fire	Congregating	Middle Daughter
☱	*Dui*	Lake	Stimulating	Youngest Daughter

ABOVE: An outline of trigram associations as translated by Master Alfred Huang.

Of the eight trigrams, only one (heaven) is full yang and only one (earth) is full yin. The rest are a blend of yin and yang with either yin or yang predominating. The following list gives the yinyang balance of each of the trigrams.

- Heaven (full yang)
- Lake (predominant yang)
- Fire (predominant yang)
- Wood / Wind (predominant yang)
- Mountain (predominant yin)
- Water (predominant yin)
- Thunder (predominant yin)
- Earth (full yin)

The lines of the trigrams act as a visual gauge of yinyang balance: you can see one element grow stronger and then weaken as the other regains control.

Each trigram has a name and a meaning based on observations of yinyang in the natural world.

THE HEXAGRAMS OF THE YEAR

You can see the bars of yin and yang move up and down in these 12 hexagrams used in ancient China to represent the months. The system shown here starts with the month of the Rat, in the middle of winter when yin is almost at full strength.

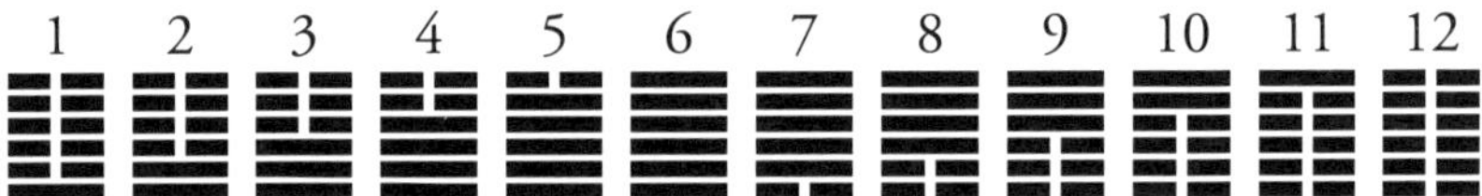

ABOVE: The 12 hexagrams of the year.

TRIGRAM ARRANGEMENTS

Historically the eight trigrams were put into various circular arrangements, which show the exchange of power between yin and yang. Remembering that a solid line is yang and a split line is yin, you can see the interplay in these notable layouts.

THE FUXI ARRANGEMENT

This arrangement of the eight trigrams shows yin and yang moving through birth, death and rebirth.

You can see that yang is at its full potential in the south, with three solid bars. Moving clockwise, yin starts to get stronger until in the north it is at its most powerful with three split bars. After this, solid yang lines start to reappear as the forces of yang make their way back to the south to return to full strength.

Note that each trigram is the direct inverse of the trigram on the opposite side of the chart (for example: east is yang-yin-yang; west is yin-yang-yin).

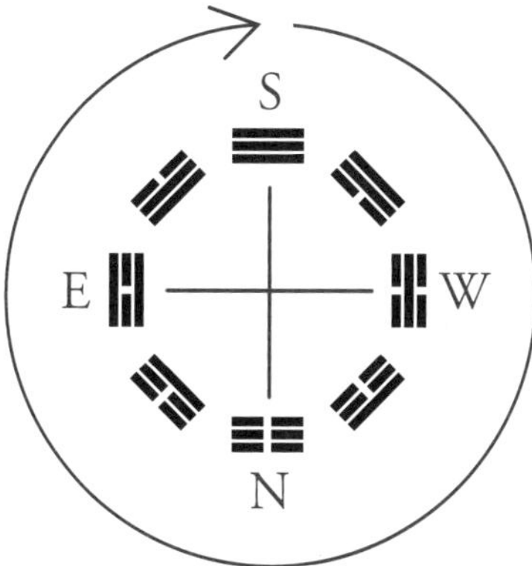

ABOVE: The Fuxi arrangement.

THE KING WEN ARRANGEMENT

The King Wen arrangement does not flow in a progress of yin and yang; instead it shows yinyang in the natural world, with fire at the top and water directly below. These two are the only direct inverses of each other in this arrangement, whereas in the Fuxi arrangement every opposite pair are inverses. In this version the progression starts in the east and moves clockwise.

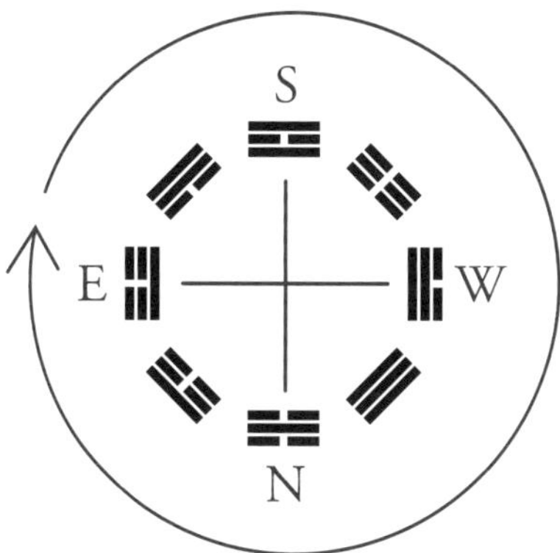

ABOVE: The King Wen arrangement.

The eight trigrams represent the rhythms of yinyang in space and time.

TRIGRAMS AS AN EARLY FORM OF WRITING

It is believed that trigrams were a precursor to Chinese writing, or that at least people used them to communicate ideas. The most often cited example of this is the apparent evolution of the water trigram into the Chinese character for water.

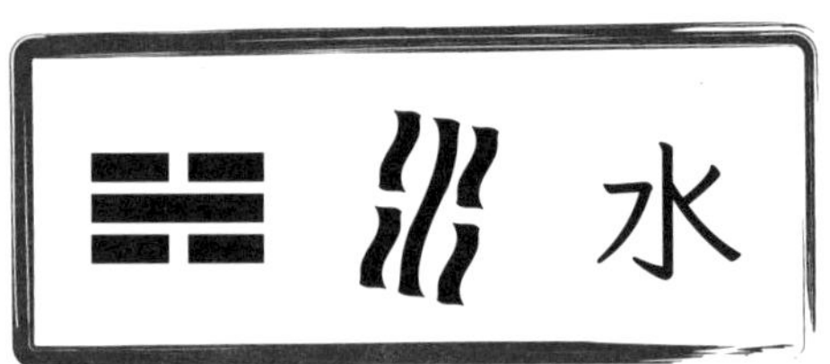

ABOVE: The water trigram (left) appears to be an early form of the ideogram for water (right).

Before the birth of Chinese writing, trigrams may have been used for communication as well as divination.

WATER AS PROTECTION

On buildings in east Asia you will sometimes find the two symbols shown in the image here. Both symbols represent water and they are used as charms to protect the building from fire.

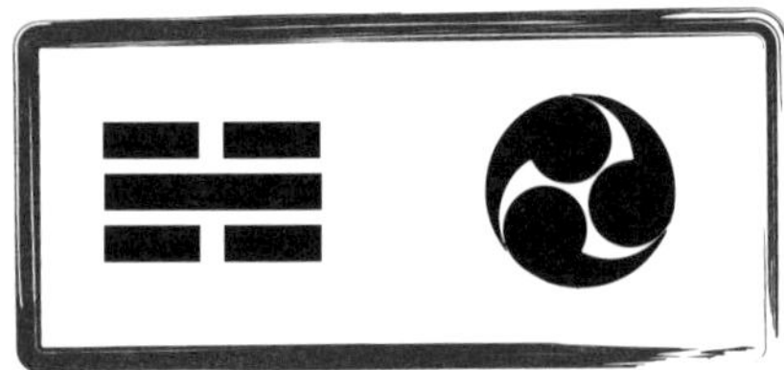

ABOVE: Symbols for water often found on buildings.

THE 64 HEXAGRAMS

As we have seen, a hexagram comprises one trigram placed on top of another and there are 64 ways in which the eight trigrams can be combined in this way, meaning that there are 64 hexagrams. Each of these hexagrams has a name and a number and they can be divided into 32 yin-dominant patterns and 32 yang-dominant patterns. The most obvious examples of yin and yang hexagrams are number 1, which is all yang, and number 2, which is all yin.

There are hexagrams that have an equal number of yin and yang lines, hexagrams that have more yin lines and hexagrams that have more yang lines. Therefore, each hexagram is either a balance of yin and yang, or is yin heavy or yang heavy.

ABOVE: Hexagram number 1 is pure yang. It is known as heaven, or *qian* in Chinese.

ABOVE: Hexagram number 2 is pure yin. It is known as earth, or *kun* in Chinese.

THE HEXAGRAM TABLE

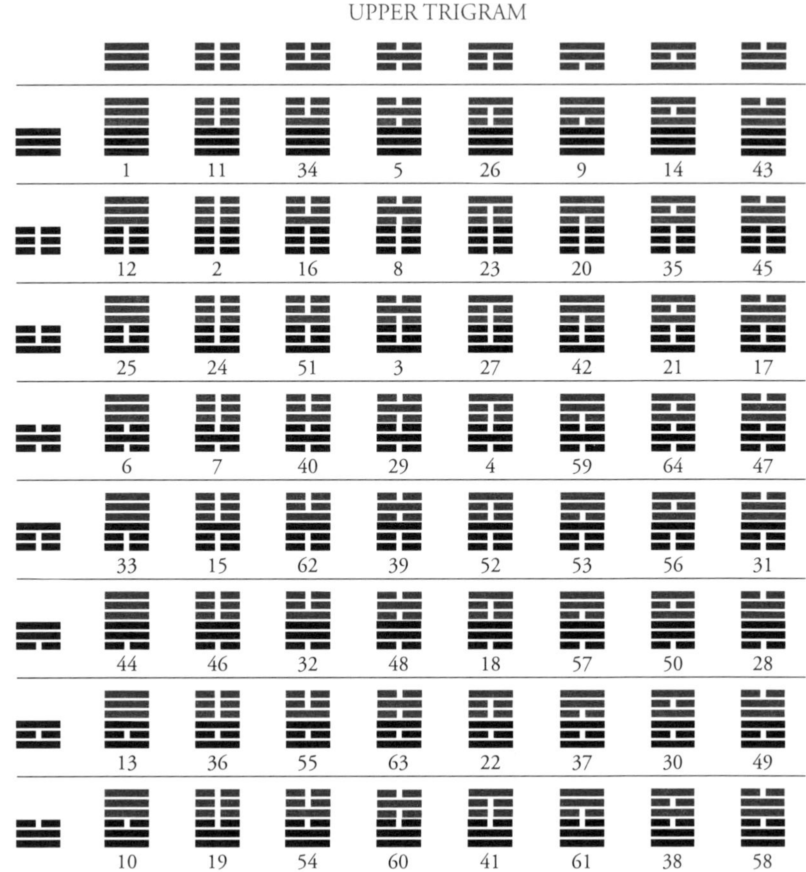

LOWER TRIGRAM \ UPPER TRIGRAM	☰	☷	☳	☵	☶	☴	☲	☱
☰	1	11	34	5	26	9	14	43
☷	12	2	16	8	23	20	35	45
☳	25	24	51	3	27	42	21	17
☵	6	7	40	29	4	59	64	47
☶	33	15	62	39	52	53	56	31
☴	44	46	32	48	18	57	50	28
☲	13	36	55	63	22	37	30	49
☱	10	19	54	60	41	61	38	58

ABOVE: The numbered hexagrams organized by upper and lower trigram.

Every book about the I-Ching should contain this standard table, which enables you to quickly discover the number of any hexagram. First match the bottom three lines of your hexagram (shown down the side of the table) to the top three lines (along the top of the table). Follow the lines to where they meet and you will find the hexagram you have cast.

For example, the hexagram with yin-yang-yin at the bottom and yang-yang-yin at the top is number 59.

The 64 hexagrams, made up of every combination of two trigrams, can be easily located on the hexagram table.

HEXAGRAM STRUCTURE

Every hexagram can be broken into sub-sections, which carry significance.

First there are the two trigrams. It is generally more auspicious for certain trigrams to be at the top or the bottom. For example, the water trigram is better at the top because water flows down, whereas the fire trigram is better at the bottom because fire travels up. If fire is at the top and water at the bottom they cannot move in their natural direction and this can cause energy to become blocked.

Next there are three two-line sections. From the bottom up, these represent earth, humans and heaven. Notice that humans are in the middle, between heaven and earth.

Finally, each individual line within each of the 64 hexagrams also has a specific meaning associated with it. Reading upward, the odd lines are yin and the even lines are yang.

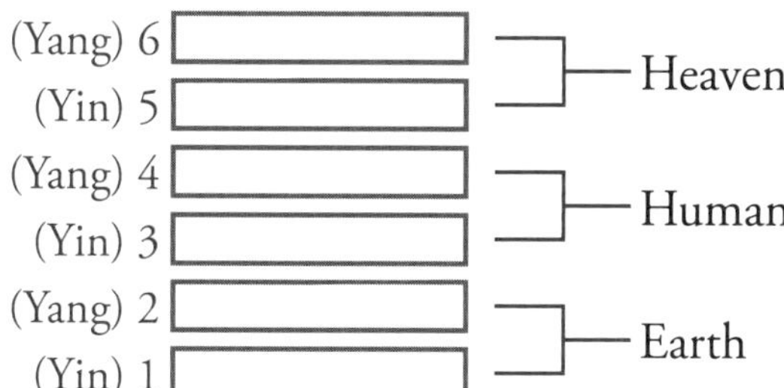

ABOVE: Hexagrams start at the bottom and finish at the top and each pair of lines is connected to earth, humans or heaven.

A hexagram is constructed and read from the bottom up – this is because energy moves upward.

THE ALTERNATIVE HEXAGRAM

There is another way to draw the hexagrams, which can often be seen in ancient Chinese manuscripts that explain the origin of the universe. In this system, the hexagram forms a circle that has three concentric rings, each of which is divided in half. The white sections represent yang and the black represent yin. The hexagram is divided down the middle so that there is a left trigram and a right trigram instead of an upper and a lower in the standard case. However, the principle remains the same – 64 combinations of six components that can be either one thing or the other.

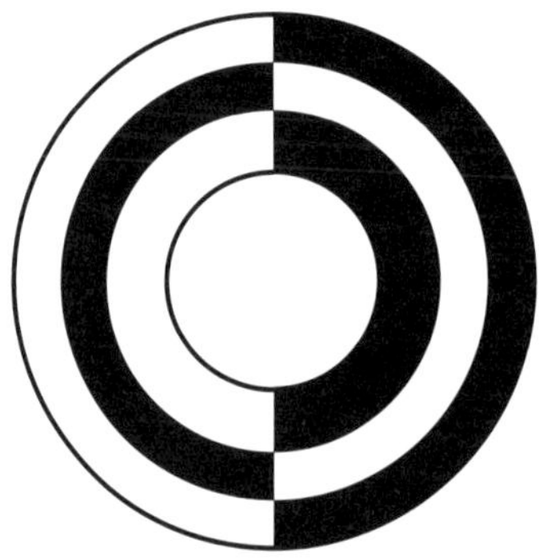

ABOVE: The alternative, circular hexagram.

☯ **The circular hexagram uses black and white sections rather than split and solid lines to represent yin and yang.**

OVERCOMING WESTERN WAYS OF THINKING

A German missionary named Richard Wilhelm brought the I-Ching back from China in the early twentieth century and since then the work has become extremely popular in both Europe and America.

However, traditional western logic can sometimes get in the way of understanding the symbolism of the I-Ching. Some trigram combinations have a more natural flow in Chinese thought. For example, a western person might see a hexagram with fire at the top and water at the bottom as a harmonious combination, because fire goes up and water goes down, whereas a Chinese person would see that this does *not* create harmony. If fire starts at the top and water at the bottom, then they are stagnant and cannot find their natural place. They have nowhere to go – and remember that the I-Ching is all about movement and change. It is more harmonious to have fire at the bottom and water at the top so that they can move through each other and find their natural positions within reality. This is just one example of how traditional Chinese thought may initially appear counter-intuitive to the western mind.

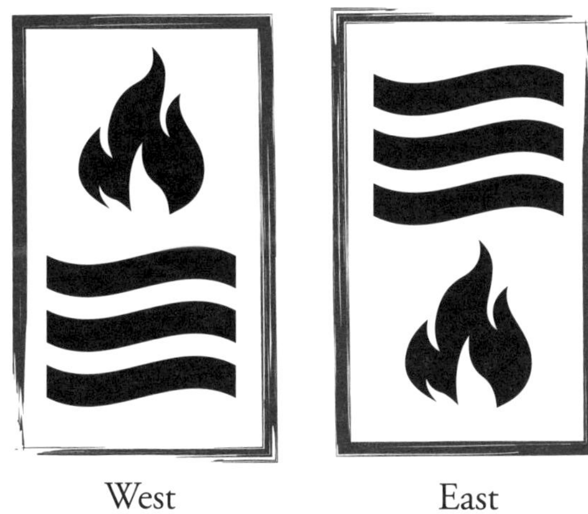

ABOVE: Western logic sees fire going up and water flowing down. Eastern logic sees water starting in the sky as clouds and fire starting on the ground as fuel.

The most harmonious hexagrams often contain the potential for movement and transformation within them.

UNDERSTANDING HUMAN EXISTENCE

From the I-Ching there are three ways to understand the universe and the existence of humans within it.

THE HUMAN EXPERIENCE

- Humans exist in the world to experience it.
- Humans experience changes.
- Humans experience uncertainty.
- Humans make decisions with the aim of improving their situation.

☯ **Humans are aware of existence and try to change their situation.**

THE COSMOLOGICAL SETTING

- All things are connected.
- Things are only defined by contrast to each other.
- Relationships between things change.
- Position within the world changes.
- Human relationships to the land change.

☯ **Yin and yang only exist through context and relationship.**

THE PRACTICAL APPLICATION OF EXISTENCE

- Humans can only ever achieve a limited understanding of the truth of the universe.
- Humans can reflect upon themselves internally and develop their nature.
- Humans understand that such development leads to progress.

☯ **Yinyang is a way for humans to understand the mystery of the universe. We try, but the mystery still remains.**

TAKING THINGS FURTHER

We have looked at the principles of I-Ching, but detailed interpretations of the hexagrams are way beyond the scope of this short chapter. There are many books and tutorials that fully explore the correct way of divination through this system and explain the hexagrams in full. It is probably best to read multiple versions of the I-Ching to appreciate the various different translations. Two good books for comparison are *The Complete I Ching* by Master Alfred Huang (Inner Traditions) and *The Original I Ching Oracle* by the Eranos I Ching Project (Watkins).

☯ **The I-Ching is a complex work which will take a great deal of dedication to master.**

WORKING WITH YINYANG:
Divine from the I-Ching

The I-Ching is an ancient system of divination which has evolved a great deal, but at its core it remains a way of understanding the movement of yinyang and how that movement creates changes within the world. At the beginning it was a way to see the universal system in progress and to ask the universe how to approach a situation, but later it became a manual for self-cultivation and internal mastery. If you try I-Ching divination and make at least a small study of the system, it will allow you to connect with the ancestors and to start to apply your own questions to the universe. Think of the I-Ching as a guiding hand to point out your position within the cosmos and the landscape.

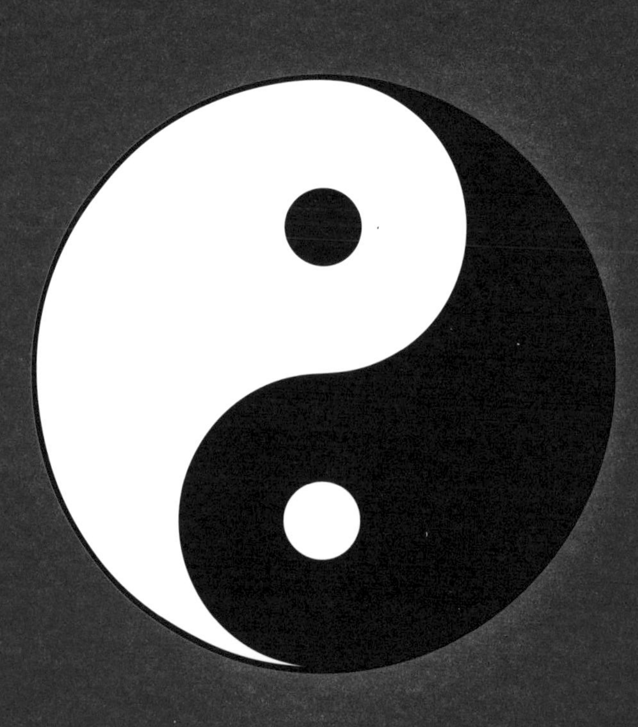

CHAPTER 10

WARFARE

WARFARE

One of the less well known aspects of yinyang theory is its application in warfare, particularly in ancient and medieval China and Japan. The Chinese military structure was based on a standing army of conscripted soldiers, much like in the Roman Empire. This system made its way to Japan, but was later replaced by the hereditary warrior class known as the samurai. The samurai continued to use many Chinese ideas, including yinyang and the Five Phases. In this chapter we will explore how the military in China and Japan used yinyang theory.

THE FOUR PILLARS OF WARFARE

There were four basic elements to warfare in old China and, subsequently, Japan:

- Strategies (権謀) – pre-planning with a solid political base
- Situational analysis (形勢) – awareness of the situation and observation of forms coming into being
- Yinyang (陰陽) – flowing with yinyang with an awareness of proper position
- Practical skills (技巧) – correct execution of strategy and technique

The fact that yinyang was considered as one of these core elements shows how highly it was regarded. It was not until the great Japanese warlords Takeda Shingen and Oda Nobunaga came to prominence in the sixteenth century that the more esoteric side of Chinese-style warfare started to wane.

☯ **Yinyang in the military was to understand the climate and the terrain including weather patterns – all of which was used to defeat the enemy.**

FORMLESS FORM

The paradoxical Asian idea of "formless form" may seem confusing at first, but it is not such a difficult concept.

An army can be lined up in columns and rows, make a wide or narrow, angled or regular shape, take a tight or loose formation. A clear structure is good and solid in the sense that each soldier will understand their role within the formation. However, it is also observable by the enemy and if something is observable then it can be exploited.

Form is important, because without form there is no structure and no tactics, and success only comes through good fortune or weight of numbers. What sets a master of war apart is their understanding of formless form. This is a well-defined, fluid internal structure that can quickly adapt to the situation, while having no discernible form from the outside. If you have no observable outward structure, others cannot predict what you will do and therefore they will find it hard to defeat you.

This principle applies not only to large armies but to individuals.

☯ **A mob without form is just a mob, but an army with no observable shape that can react to commands in an instant has mastered "formless form".**

SUBSTANTIAL AND INSUBSTANTIAL

The concept of substantial and insubstantial, said as *xushi* in Chinese and *kyojitsu* in Japanese, is the understanding of truth and deception and the relationship between yourself and the enemy. Warfare is about making the enemy think you are strong where you are weak and weak where you are strong. It is to sow doubt in the enemy's mind, to make them question if what you are presenting is a truth or a lie. Each side is trying to tempt the enemy to attack where they are strongest and identify and attack where the enemy is weakest.

The ancient Chinese battle of Red Cliffs is often given as an example of this concept in action. An army that was running low on equipment was facing an overwhelming force who were well equipped, so their tactician devised a plan. On a morning of heavy fog he sent out many boats stuffed full of dummy soldiers made of straw. The enemy, seeing the war boats approach in the fog, shot volley after volley of arrows, and after some time the boats retreated. The arrows were plucked undamaged from the straw and redistributed among the allied archers so that they were equipped for the real battle at the expense of their opponents.

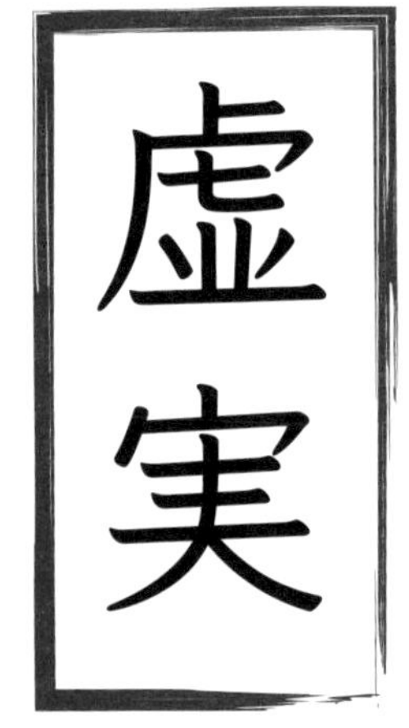

ABOVE: The Chinese characters for *xushi*, the idea of substantial and insubstantial.

In this example, the insubstantial (fake soldiers) was presented as substantial (an attack), with the result that the enemy lost something substantial (arrows) and were left in an insubstantial state (with fewer arrows). Remember, what is presented to you is often not the truth.

☯ **Warfare is a battle of deception in which each side hides their own weaknesses while searching for those of their enemy.**

YINYANG IN JAPAN

As well as having their native Shinto religion, the Japanese were heavily influenced by traditions imported from China such as Buddhism, Confucianism and, not least, Daoism. Known in Japanese as *dokyo*, Daoism was the foundation of *onmyodo*, "the way of yinyang". In Japanese, yinyang becomes *in-yo*. The ideograms are the same and so is the philosophy. Yinyang permeated all areas of society, including the military class. For example, when *yabusame* mounted archers galloped down the field toward their target, they screamed "*in-yo*, *in-yo*, *in-yo*" ("yinyang, yinyang, yinyang").

The adoption of Daoism created a problem for the Japanese in that it gave them two creation myths. There was the native version in which the islands of Japan were formed from drops of water from a jewelled spear carried by the god and goddess Izanagi and Izanami, and then there was the Daoist version in which the world was created through the movement of yin and yang. Both origin stories were told side by side throughout Japanese history.

☯ Yinyang was as influential in Japan as in China.

THE ENERGY OF WAR

Male yang (*yo*) energy is fierce. Therefore, when samurai went to battle they stepped off with the left leg, the leg of yang, and they also forbade their wives from seeing them off at the gate for fear that female yin (*in*) energy would dampen their aggression.

☯ War is the domain of yang energy and it is predominantly men who are warriors. However, there are some examples of female fighters in Japan.

SAMURAI MILITARY EQUIPMENT

For the samurai, yinyang energy was an important consideration not only in military strategy but also in equipment such as helmets, horses and war curtains.

HELMETS

The characteristic gold or silver segments sometimes found at the top of a samurai helmet represent different aspects of yinyang.

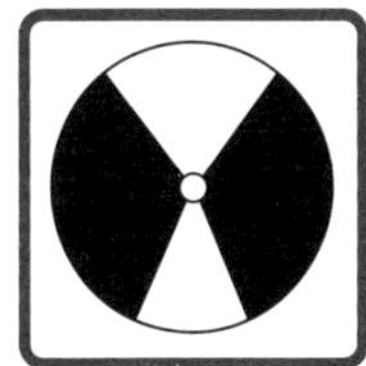
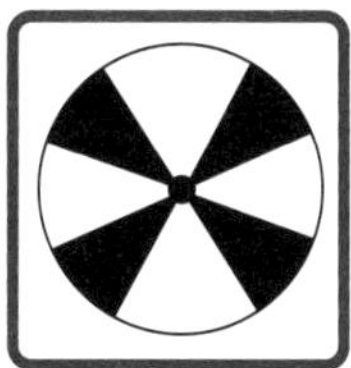
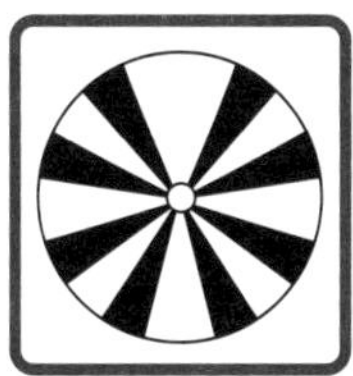

ABOVE: Samurai helmet bowls as seen from above, with the white areas representing gold or silver segments.

- A helmet with two segments is called a *nihojiro* (二方白). It is considered to be equal in yin and yang.

- A helmet with four segments is called a *shihojiro* (四方白). It is a helmet of yin power.

- A helmet with eight segments is called a *happojiro* (八方白). It is a helmet of yang power.

HORSES

A samurai's horse had to meet the normal standards of strength, stamina, speed and courage, but it also had to be the right colour. This is because a horse was deemed to be of a certain element, be it earth, fire, metal, water or wood, depending on its colour – a system based on Five Phase theory (see chapter 16). If a samurai's own element was in a phase of destruction in relation to the horse's element, then it was not the horse for him. He would have to find a horse of an element that was in a creative relationship to his element so that positive energy would flow through him and the horse.

Samurai would also send horses of ill omen to the enemy as a form of ritual attack magic.

The following poem from the *Book of Samurai* series explains which horse colour is associated with which element.

芦青木栗毛雲雀火鹿粕土月瓦金黒ニ毛ハ水

"Grey and bluish-black horses are of wood; chestnut and yellowish dapple with blackish mane and tail are of fire; bay and roan are of earth; palomino and buckskin are of metal; and black and sa-me *are of water."*

SAME DIFFERENCE

The Japanese word sa-me *(pronounced "san-may") refers to horses that are known as "double dilutes" in English. These are horses that have two copies of the cream gene. They have pale cream hair with pink skin showing through, giving slight variations of tone.*

WAR CURTAINS

Samurai armies who were in the field would erect curtain walls to partition different areas. The name for the samurai government is the *bakufu* (幕府), "government within the curtain", a term which comes from the use of cloth enclosures to section off a command centre. These curtains were in pairs, and they were named yin and yang curtains.

Traditional Japanese warships were wooden and surrounded by shield boards. Outside of these shields was a double-layered set of curtains, which reached down the sides of the ship and touched the water's surface. These often carried clan markings. The outside layer was the yang curtain, while the inside layer was the yin curtain.

☯ **Yinyang infused many items in a samurai warrior's armoury. Those discussed above are just a few examples.**

SAMURAI CUSTOMS

The following is a selection of particular samurai customs and practices influenced by yinyang.

CALMING THE TROOPS

Samurai leaders would order a rowdy army to sit down. Sitting is associated with yin, which is more calming than the warlike yang, the element of standing.

LAYING OUT THE DEAD

On a battlefield or after a raid, bodies had to be laid out correctly. Men were laid on their backs, which is a yang position because it faces the sky; women were laid on their fronts, which is a yin position because it faces the earth.

TYING KNOTS

In samurai culture, a knot that tied to the left was yang and one that tied to the right was yin. Even the handheld torches they used had to have the correct knots on them. These were used by spies as secret identifying marks so that they could recognize other spies on their side.

Yinyang extended to the weave of fabrics, which were divided into yin and yang directions – clothes for death and clothes for life.

TRAVELLING BY ROAD

In old Japan different parts of a road were associated with yin or yang. At certain times of the day, samurai would walk along the middle of the road, because it had the *chi* of yang. However, at a certain hour they would move over to the side of the road, because the *chi* of the road was reversed.

☯ **The samurai had a deep relationship with yinyang and they relied on it to shape their warrior culture.**

THE SHINOBI

Within every samurai army were shadowy figures known as shinobi, the commando-spies of the East. The shinobi are better known today as ninja. Dealing with sabotage, subterfuge, espionage and all things underhanded, they operated separately from the main army but were still a vital part of the samurai war machine. One way in which they did not differ from conventional troops was in their strict adherence to the principles of yinyang.

LOST MEANINGS

Trying to make sense of old Chinese and Japanese scrolls is fascinating, but can be frustrating when meanings prove hard to pin down. One example comes in the seventeenth-century shinobi scroll written by Hattori Doson. He uses two intriguing terms: insei *(陰盛), meaning "yin and prosperous", and* yokyo *(陽虚), meaning "yang and insubstantial". However, the explanation of these terms was passed down only by oral tradition and has been lost. The rest of the scroll is translated in* Samurai and Ninja *by Antony Cummins (Tuttle, 2015).*

YIN AND YANG SHINOBI ARTS

The tasks of the shinobi were divided into the aspects of yin and yang (*in* and *yo* in Japanese). Yin-shinobi was to use the dark of night to creep about. Yang-shinobi was to operate in plain sight – where people could see the agent but did not know they were on a secret mission.

> *"The basic principle of* shinobi no jutsu *contains* in-nin *and* yo-nin *at its root, but it diversifies itself into ever-changing and countless styles, like the leaves and branches of a tree, so much so that not everything can be described here."*
>
> *The Book of Ninja* by Antony Cummins and Yoshie Minami (Watkins, 2013)

The combination of yin and yang created endless skill sets for the shinobi, just like it creates the endless universe. For example, a shinobi might use yin skills to infiltrate under cover of darkness. Then, once within the enemy walls, they would change to the aspect of yang – perhaps by assuming the disguise of a guard or a messenger in order to get through a check point without arousing suspicion. They might then return to the aspect of yin and press on to achieve their goal. Part of the skill of the shinobi was knowing when to creep and when to bluff.

USING YINYANG AS A DISGUISE

Japan, just like China, had wandering yinyang diviners who would travel around the country selling their skills. The shinobi often disguised themselves as these itinerant specialists in yinyang to move freely around enemy territory. So yinyang could be used not only as a method but a disguise.

THE YINYANG MINDSET OF THE SHINOBI

A shinobi's body was yin, which meant it was passive and prepared for death, but their mind was yang – strong and warlike. They cared nothing for the risk to their own bodies, but their aggressive mindset protected them from harm.

SUPERSTITIONS

Out on a mission, the shinobi would be guided by signs and omens, such as the pattern made by the leaves in their tea, or the shape of a plume of incense smoke. Yinyang played an important part in this. For example, a yin animal coming from a yin direction was bad luck, whereas a yang animal coming from a yang direction was good luck.

☯ **Switching seamlessly between overt and covert operations, the shadowy shinobi were the ultimate yinyang warriors.**

SHINOBI SKILLS FEATURING YINYANG

The following is a list of shinobi skills that include the terms yin and yang, or in *and* yo. *They were recorded by the eighteenth-century military historian Chikamatsu Shigenori.*

- In yo shinobi no daiji *(*陰陽忍之大事*) – the principle of yinyang shinobi*
- In yo tomoni majiwaru koto *(*陰陽倶錯事*) – concerning yin and yang*
- Yo maku no koto *(*陽幕之事*) – the art of yang war curtains*
- Yo shinobi no koto *(*陽忍之事*) – the art of yang shinobi*

WORKING WITH YINYANG

Follow the rhythms of yinyang to succeed

We are not all soldiers, but sometimes we have to fight to achieve our goals, and this may pit us against an opponent we have to overcome. You can use the skills of yinyang to gain the upper hand. Be like the shinobi: know when to practise yin-shinobi – working under cover of darkness – and when to practise yang-shinobi – operating in plain sight. Be like the samurai general: hide your weaknesses, tempt your opponent to attack your strengths, probe for their weaknesses. If we follow its rhythms, yinyang will show us the way to gain victory.

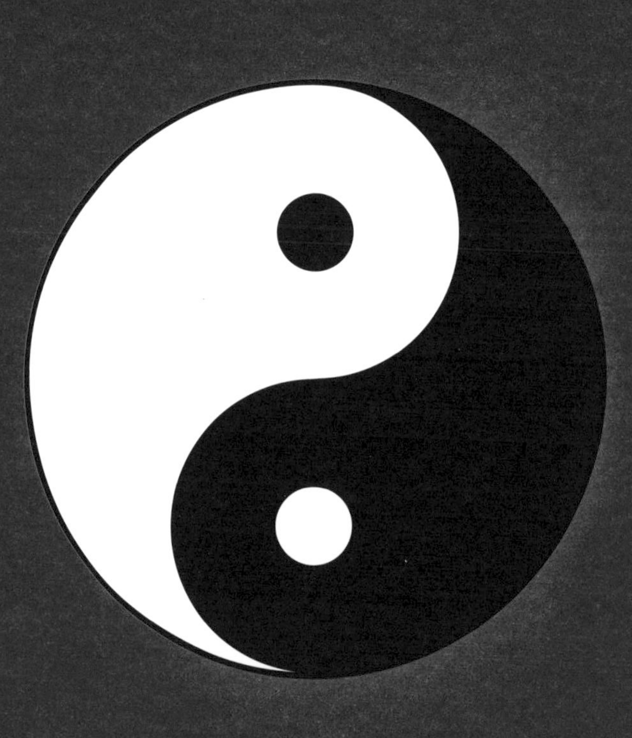

CHAPTER 11

MEASURING TIME AND SPACE

MEASURING TIME AND SPACE

The point of yinyang is to follow the patterns of the world and find the position within both the landscape and society that benefits us the most, while avoiding those places and situations that will damage us. Yinyang is about riding the waves of the world so that we come out on top. In this chapter we will look at the systems that enable us to understand our position within time and space. They may seem somewhat abstract, but they are fundamental in all subjects relating to yinyang, from Traditional Chinese Medicine to the military arts of the East.

THE FOUR CARDINAL DIRECTIONS

As discussed in chapter 2, the basic directions of north, east, south and west and the centre are each connected to one of the Five Phases. They are also associated with a colour and are guarded by symbolic creatures that have a prominent position in Chinese culture. The table opposite summarizes these associations.

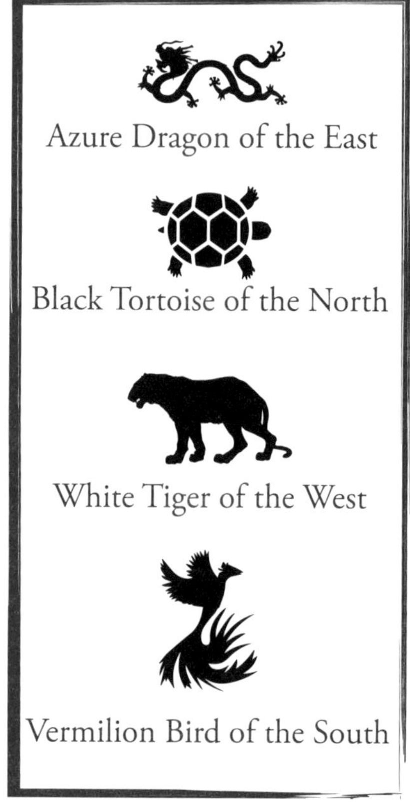

RIGHT: The symbolic animals that guard the four cardinal points on the horizon (these are not to be confused with the animals of the zodiac).

THE CARDINAL POINTS AND THEIR ATTRIBUTES			
DIRECTION	PHASE	COLOUR	SYMBOL
Centre	Earth	Yellow / Gold	Golden dragon
South	Fire	Red	Red bird
East	Wood	Light blue-green	Light blue-green dragon
North	Water	Black	Black tortoise
West	Metal	White	White tiger

Each cardinal direction, and the centre, is associated with one of the Five Phases and is represented by a colour and an animal.

HOW DRAGONS WENT EXTINCT

In ancient times there were officials assigned to each of the four directions (and also a fifth for the earth at the centre). Their task was to ensure that the correct rituals were performed for the animal associated with each direction and to placate the gods of those areas. However, legend has it that one day the minister responsible for the dragons failed in his duty and as a consequence dragons either fled the area or died out. That is why to this day you will never see a dragon.

THE 12 EARTHLY BRANCHES

The Chinese observed the star constellation known as Ursa Major (the Great Bear) and depending on which way it was pointing they could identify 12 separate directions, which they called the 12 Earthly Branches (十二支). Each named after an animal, they are the main sections of the zodiac. As well as being the units into which the ancient Chinese broke up the horizon and the day, they are fundamental to understanding many other aspects of east Asian thought.

The following table itemizes the 12 Earthly Branches, what they stand for and how they are represented.

THE 12 EARTHLY BRANCHES AND THEIR ASSOCIATIONS					
IDEOGRAM	ANIMAL	APPROXIMATE TIME	DEGREES	APPROXIMATE DIRECTION	ELEMENT
子	Rat	11pm–1am	0 or 360°	North	Water
丑	Ox	1am–3am	30°	NEbN	Earth
寅	Tiger	3am–5am	60°	NEbE	Wood
卯	Hare	5am–7am	90°	East	Wood
辰	Dragon	7am–9am	120°	SEbE	Earth
巳	Snake	9am–11am	150°	SEbS	Fire

THE 12 EARTHLY BRANCHES AND THEIR ASSOCIATIONS					
IDEOGRAM	ANIMAL	APPROXIMATE TIME	DEGREES	APPROXIMATE DIRECTION	ELEMENT
午	Horse	11am–1pm	180°	South	Fire
未	Ram	1pm–3pm	210°	SWbS	Earth
申	Monkey	3pm–5pm	240°	SWbW	Metal
酉	Cockerel	5pm–7pm	270°	West	Metal
戌	Dog	7pm–9pm	300°	NWbW	Earth
亥	Boar	9pm–11pm	330°	NWbN	Water

Originally the moon was used to mark months, because it is easy to observe the cycle of the moon. This is known as a lunar month. However, the lunar cycle varies between 27 and 29 days, so for ease the Chinese divided the months into two types, "small months" of 29 days and "long months" of 30 days, to fit the calendar better to the full year. However, this did not equate exactly to the 365.25 days it takes the earth to orbit the sun, so at times they had to make adjustments to add or deduct days.

☯ The 12 Earthly Branches laid the foundations for many Chinese systems and skills.

THE 10 HEAVENLY STEMS

The 10 Heavenly (or Celestial) Stems was the original dating system of the Chinese. For example, the ancient Chinese 10-day week was based on the Heavenly Stems. Originally named after Chinese rulers from ancient times, they fell out of favour and were largely replaced by the 12 Earthly Branches. However, they continued to influence many traditional Asian practices.

The following table gives an overview of the 10 Heavenly Stems.

THE 10 HEAVENLY STEMS						
NUMBER	ELEMENT (CYCLE OF CREATION)	CHINESE NAME	JAPANESE NAME	STEM	STATUS	YINYANG
1	Wood	*Jia*	*Kinoe*	甲	Greater	Yang
2	Wood	*Yi*	*Kinoto*	乙	Lesser	Yin
3	Fire	*Bing*	*Hinoe*	丙	Greater	Yang
4	Fire	*Ding*	*Hinoto*	丁	Lesser	Yin
5	Earth	*Wu*	*Tsuchinoe*	戊	Greater	Yang
6	Earth	*Ji*	*Tsuchinoto*	己	Lesser	Yin

THE 10 HEAVENLY STEMS						
NUMBER	ELEMENT (CYCLE OF CREATION)	CHINESE NAME	JAPANESE NAME	STEM	STATUS	YINYANG
7	Metal	*Geng*	*Kanoe*	庚	Greater	Yang
8	Metal	*Xin*	*Kanoto*	辛	Lesser	Yin
9	Water	*Ren*	*Mizunoe*	壬	Greater	Yang
10	Water	*Gui*	*Mizunoto*	癸	Lesser	Yin

The Heavenly Stems are often labelled as either "big brother" (兄) or "little brother" (弟), corresponding to the "greater" and "lesser" status classifications in the table. As you will see from the table, the greater stems are yang and the lesser stems are yin. An elder brother is considered to be more vigorous (and therefore more yang) than a younger brother. Each element has a greater and a lesser phase, which are each represented by one of the stems.

These waxing and waning stages of each of the Five Phases can be described in natural terms as follows:

- **Wood** – Trees burst forth with blossom (yang) before becoming laden with fruit (yin).
- **Fire** – An inferno blazes (yang) but eventually dies down (yin).
- **Earth** – Soil gives life to plants (yang), but can erode to become thin and lifeless (yin).

- **Metal** – A gleaming iron axe (yang) can rust and become blunt (yin).
- **Water** – A torrential downpour (yang) dies out into a few last droplets (yin).

THE JOURNEY OF LIFE

The 10 Heavenly Stems can also be used to plot the journey of a human life, as described in the table below.

THE 10 STAGES OF HUMAN LIFE		
STEM	PERIOD	DESCRIPTION
1	Birth	Coming into the world
2	Nursing	State of vulnerability
3	Toddler	Rapid growth
4	Youth	Slower continual growth
5	Prime	Physical strength
6	Middle age	Peak state
7	Ageing	Decline from strength
8	Twilight years	From weak to just before death

THE 10 STAGES OF HUMAN LIFE		
STEM	PERIOD	DESCRIPTION
9	Death	Departure of *chi*
10	Decay	Generation of *chi* from the body after death

The animals of the four directions, the 12 Earthly Branches and the 10 Heavenly Stems interact to create a complex network of ways to measure the natural world. It is important to understand them individually before considering how they relate to each other.

THE 24 SOLAR TERMS

Another traditional Chinese way to measure the year was called the 24 Solar Terms (二十四節気), points in the calendar that marked the passage of the seasons in terms of weather and agriculture. Farming was one of the primary concerns in the ancient world, where life often depended on a successful harvest:

1. Start of spring (立春)
2. Rain water (雨水)
3. Awakening of the insects (啓蟄)
4. Spring equinox (春分)
5. Pure brightness (清明)
6. Grain rain (穀雨)
7. Start of summer (立夏)
8. Sprouting grain (小満)

9 Grain forms ears (芒種)

10 Summer solstice (夏至)

11 Minor heat (小暑)

12 Major heat (大暑)

13 Start of autumn (立秋)

14 Limit of heat (処暑)

15 White dew (白露)

16 Autumnal equinox (秋分)

17 Cold dew (寒露)

18 Descent of the frost (霜降)

19 Start of winter (立冬)

20 Minor snow (小雪)

21 Major snow (大雪)

22 Winter solstice (冬至)

23 Minor cold (小寒)

24 Major cold (大寒)

☯ The 24 Solar Terms map out the year in terms of the farming seasons. In the old days, people did not need to know the date so much as they needed to understand how to grow food.

WORKING WITH YINYANG:
Observe customs and festivals to honour the changing year

Today many of us live urban lives in which we keep constant track of the time and date, but may forget about the seasons and the traditional calendar. Try to focus more on how the weather and landscape are constantly changing about you as each year progresses and how this affects plants and wildlife. Understand that as the seasons change, yin and yang will move through phases of power and decline. Look at how the changing year impacts on your local environment and consider participating in festivals, celebrations of solar events, local customs and so on to mark the passing of time.

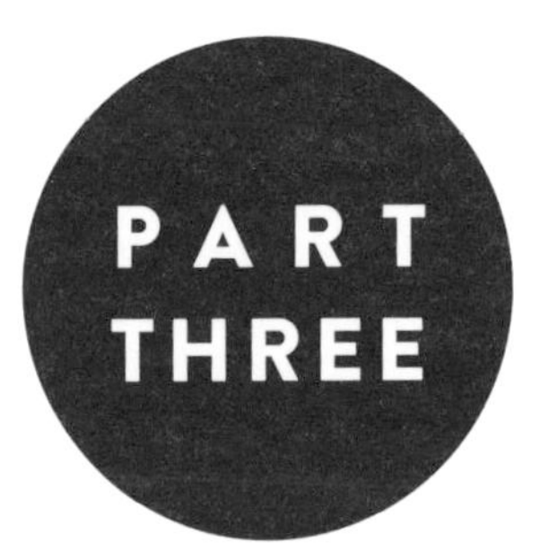

BRINGING YINYANG INTO YOUR LIFE

In the first two parts of this book we looked at the concept of yinyang and how it evolved. Now we will see how it is actually used. How did the people of ancient China interact with it and how can you adjust your own life to the concept of yinyang? As well as being a way to understand the universe and the world we live in, yinyang is also a system that enables us to get the most out of our existence. We can all learn how to live in alignment with nature and follow the Way to provide a better life for ourselves and our family.

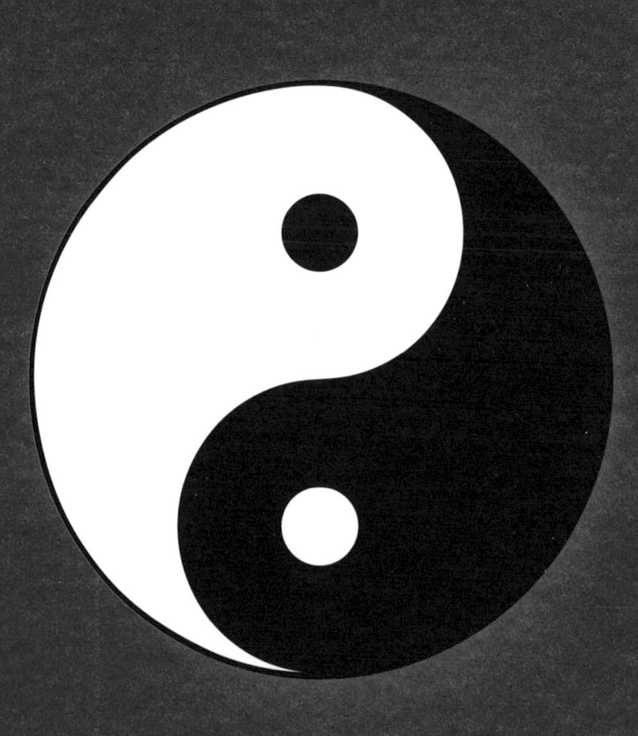

CHAPTER 12

FINDING THE WAY

FINDING THE WAY

Having been introduced to the Dao or Way in chapter 5, now it is time to delve more deeply into the concept. This will help you understand how yinyang works at its basic level and how you can use it to ride the waves of the universe and live in a more fruitful manner. It is important to understand not only what we know about the Way, but also what we do not – and the problems that overestimating our knowledge can cause.

THE WAY AND THE WAY

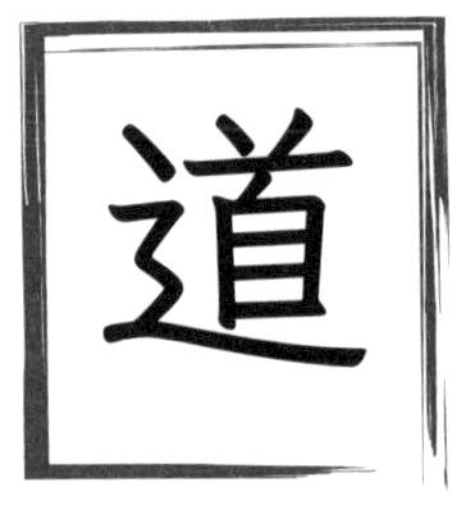

ABOVE: The ideogram for the Dao.

The Chinese term Dao (道) has two meanings; they are connected but it is important to understand the difference. In its primary sense it is the laws of the universe which underpin the reality of existence. This we refer to as the "Way", with a capital "W". Secondly it refers to a path that a human can take to live in harmony with the Way, such as the way of tea, the way of calligraphy, the way of the warrior, and so on. This has a lower-case "w".

The two senses of the Dao may have arisen as different schools developed divergent theories. Daoism is based on the notion of the Way as the all-encompassing nature of the universe, whereas Confucianism took the more human-centric view that it represented a way that a person acts and the path that they follow. To further confuse matters, Buddhism also uses the term to mean the path to enlightenment through the teachings of Buddha.

The ideogram used for the Dao represents the head of a person wearing a cowl and walking down a winding path with a cane, probing the way ahead. This accommodates both main senses of the term – as a conventional "path" or "way" and as the spiritual "Way" laid out by heaven. The "Great Path" (大道) is there to guide us so that we do not have to wander aimlessly but can follow the intention of the universe.

The "Way" means the laws of the universe; a "way" is a path or art that if followed correctly helps us to live in harmony with the Way.

FORMS OF THE DAO

The ideogram for the Dao is used on its own to represent the Way and in combination with other ideograms to represent various ways. The following are the main examples.

天道
Tiandao
The way of heaven

To understand the celestial bodies and patterns in the sky. This is to study the heavens in a physical, astronomical sense rather than heaven in a philosophical, spiritual sense.

人道
Rendao
The way of humans

The rituals, systems and concepts attributed to humankind.

地道
Didao
The way of earth

An understanding of nature and the patterns of the world.

Everything starts with the Way, but the human mind seeks to break things down into more manageable ways.

ONE WAY SYSTEM

Despite our tendency to break everything down into categories, we need to understand that the world is not a collection of separate things. There is no end of one thing and start of another; all things are states of *chi* which have come together through a mixing of yin and yang, a movement that comes from the Way. Therefore, all things are connected. There is simply no separation between each of us and everything else and it is only our own limited observation that stops us from understanding this essential truth.

☯ **Everything is connected. This idea is conveyed in an alternative term for the Dao, which is *taiyi* (太一) – "the great oneness".**

THE WAY IS FORMLESS

The Way has no observable form, yet it still has an effect on the physical world. The laws of nature have no form, mathematics has no form, the principles of physics have no form and electricity has no form, yet all of them make a difference. The Way is the same but on a cosmic level.

☯ **The Way has no form yet was here before the universe. It is here now, it binds all things and it can be interacted with, yet it remains formless and unobservable.**

BEFORE TIME AND SPACE THERE WAS THE WAY

The state before the universe had no time, no matter, no location and no emptiness, but it held the Way because the Way was not born and will not die (birth and death being a product of time). There can be a "before" the universe, because time has only existed for as long as the universe has existed. In that "before" was only the Way, the essence of all possibility of future life (even though the future was not yet a concept).

There is no need to understand this at a logical level, because it cannot be understood logically. We have entered into a place beyond human comprehension; there are no facts or statistics to define the pre-universe. The Way that can be named is not the Way, because describing something requires a "something" to describe.

Before the universe there was no "something", nor was there a "nothing". There was only the Way.

THE WAY THAT CAN BE NAMED IS NOT THE WAY

"The Dao that can be named is not the real Dao, while the name that can be named is not the real name."

Lao Tzu's famous opening to the Dao De Jing, which we touched upon earlier in the book, is worth examining more deeply.

If you discuss the Way as if you understand it, you are not talking about the actual Way; you are giving your interpretation of it. The Way is the incomprehensible source of all creation. To claim that you understand the Way would be as outlandish as a scientist promising to tell you every secret of the universe. The simple fact is that humans do not know what is beyond our existence.

What we can do is use analogy and metaphor to communicate an interpretation of the Way. Lao Tzu is not saying that we *cannot* talk about the Way. In fact, the whole point of the Dao De Jing is that it *does* talk about the Way, and every Daoist since Lao Tzu has also talked about the Way. The whole point of Daoism and of yinyang theory is to observe the Way in action, to discuss it and then engage with it even if our view is limited by the lens of human understanding.

The Way cannot be defined or understood, but it can be observed in action and discussed through analogy.

THE WAY CANNOT PRODUCE WITHOUT MOVEMENT

Before the universe existed, the Way did not create. Without the laws of physics, without time, without space, without the concept of nothing, there is no movement and no such thing as context or comparison. It was only through the movement, the division and the generation of yinyang that the "process" started. Therefore, while the Way is the source of the laws of nature, yinyang is the inertia that brings about all creation.

☯ **The division of yin and yang created the first context and state of comparison. That was the start of me and you as an idea.**

THE WAY IS LIMITLESS

All things spring from the Way and the movement of yinyang. The earth holds more than enough for everyone to lead a happy and fulfilled life. If everyone followed the correct way of living, taking only what they needed to live in relative comfort, then the earth would be a paradise and all people would be content.

However, this does not mean that it is other people's actions that stop us from leading a fruitful and ample life. Quite the reverse – it is the actions of each human that either connect them to or disconnect them from the Way, thereby bringing about their good or bad situation. It is through proper living and connection with the Way that abundance follows.

☯ **A sense that something is wrong in our life tells us that we have strayed from the Way and need to find it again.**

KARMIC DEBT

This is a good point to explain why Daoism and Buddhism are often studied together in Asia. The Way says that there is enough for all people to live a good and happy life, but we know that sometimes good things happen to bad people and bad things happen to good people. Buddhism explains this through the concept of karmic debt, which is like a tally of all the negative actions a person has committed through living incorrectly. When a person acts in accordance with the Way – both in the Buddhist and the Daoist sense of the term – they do not add to their karmic debt, but they may have old debt that still has to be paid off. This can take lifetimes, but do not be disheartened. It is always best to stay on the path so that you do not have to suffer more in the future.

THE "TEN THOUSAND THINGS"

A common idea in Chinese thought is *wanwu* (萬物), which means "ten thousand things". This term encompasses everything observable and identifiable in the known universe. It does not refer simply to concrete objects but also includes abstract emotions and ideas – anything that is subjectively experienced within time and space.

☯ **The term "ten thousand things" is a common saying in many books on Asia. It means "all of creation".**

SHIFTING CATEGORIES

The idea that everything in the world can be classified according to its relationship with yinyang is known as *lei* (類). It is a vastly complex system and is akin to a directory of yinyang.

Remember that yin and yang are relative, and so *lei* is full of "moving categorizations". For example, snow is yin because it is cold and yin is cold. But when snow is understood as a part of heaven because it comes from the sky it is yang, because heaven is yang. Yinyang is fluid and so is *lei*.

☯ Yin and yang are relative, so everything changes category according to context.

WORKING WITH YINYANG:
Have faith in the Way

It is important to truly get to grips with the Way. Even if we know it cannot be understood, what we can gain from our human interpretation of it helps us live a better life. Knowing that the Way is flowing through the universe, that it was there before time and space but that it is also present at all times and in all places, will set you on the right path from the start. This will also help you not to get disheartened when life seems to throw troubles your way. Keep following the path, have faith in it, and it will lead you through good times and bad.

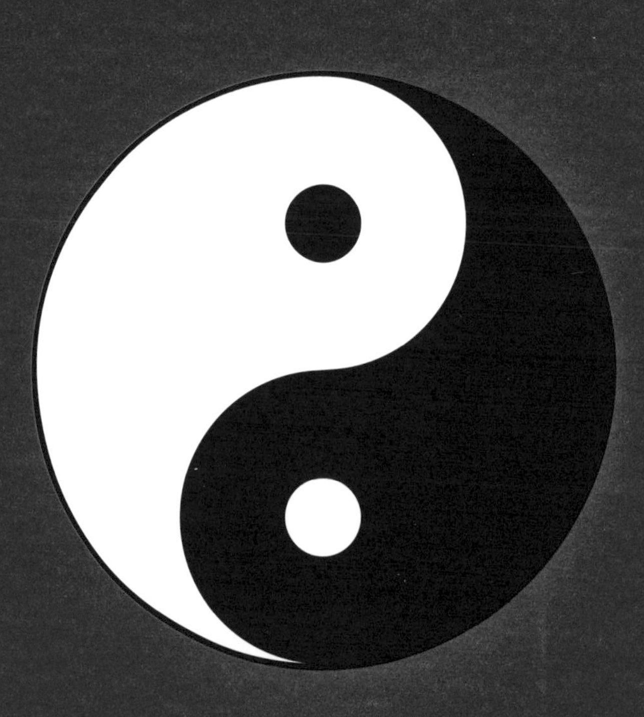

CHAPTER 13

UNDERSTANDING *CHI*

UNDERSTANDING *CHI*

Knowing that the Dao is outside of space and time and that it generates movement through yinyang brings us to the idea of *chi*, the "electricity", divine spark and power of all creation. If the Dao is the laws of the universe, its patterns and plans, and yinyang its two balancing parts, then *chi* is the charge that runs through all things and brings everything to life. This chapter will outline the nature of *chi* and help you prepare to harness its benefits – because, before you can use *chi*, you must understand it.

WHAT IS *CHI*?

Chi is extremely difficult to describe; it is unobservable, it is unproven, it is all-encompassing, it is ever-changing. There are many analogies for *chi* and various ways to understand it. *Chi* is in everything, it is everything. It is the connecting force of all existence without which the universe would break up and cease to exist. Think of *chi* as the energy of the universe, flowing through the whole of creation: it pulsates, it speeds up, it slows down, it reforms, it dissipates, and it goes through various stages of power – all of which makes for a dynamic existence. *Chi* is shaped by the things it inhabits but it also shapes the universe. There are contradictions and unanswerable questions within *chi* that Chinese thinkers have been trying to resolve for millennia. Remember, these ideas did not come from a single source; they developed through the interaction of many schools and therefore there are some points of contest.

☯ ***Chi* is the energy that holds together the "ten thousand things" of creation.**

THE PROBLEM OF TIME

Which came first: the movement of yinyang which generated chi, *or the arrival of* chi *which moved the two parts of yinyang? We will always run into problems if we view this process from a modern, linear perspective. Instead, try to see things like the ancient Chinese did – as a constantly evolving state.*

THE IDEOGRAM FOR *CHI*

The ideogram that represents *chi* (氣 or 気) consists of steam or vapour rising from a bowl of rice. This gives the sense of *chi* as an energy that emanates from something and rises above it. The ideogram may originally have been used as a verb – to represent the action of emanation and rising rather than the steam itself.

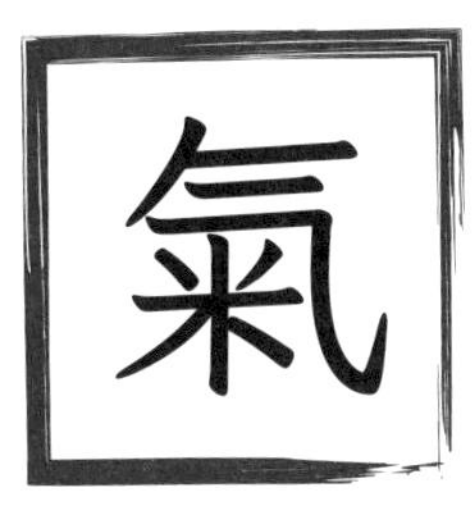

ABOVE: The ideogram for *chi* has evolved and has multiple forms. However, this is the most common version.

You will find the ideogram transcribed in one of three ways:

- *Ch'i* (or *chi*)
- *Qi*
- *Ki* (Japanese)

All three represent the same idea. Only the spelling and pronunciation vary. The apostrophe is technically correct, but in modern usage is often dropped. Strictly speaking, the Chinese version of the word is pronounced "kuh-ee", whereas the Japanese is pronounced "kee", but this is a subtle distinction and "kee" is an acceptable pronunciation for all forms.

Be careful not to confuse *chi* (氣) when written as *qi* (氣) with a separate term written the same way. This other *qi* uses a different ideogram (器) and in the context of yinyang means "tangible things", meaning things that are observable in the universe. So *qi* can mean either the energy of life (氣) or the tangible things created by the energy of life (器).

☯ ***Chi* rises and produces a "smoky" edge around any living thing.**

THE SIX FORMS OF *CHI*

Originally *chi* was a separate entity outside of yinyang in some of the earliest schools of thought. There were six aspects to it:

- Cold (yin)
- Heat (yang)
- Wind
- Rain
- Darkness
- Light

The original ideograms for dark and bright are different from the ideograms for yin and yang in the six forms of *chi*, while yin and yang are seen as cold and heat and as aspects of the weather.

From these six qualities, all other sub-divisions were created: the five tastes, the five colours, the five notes, the six diseases, and so on. These six types of *chi* were the basis for all life.

☯ **For early cultures, light and dark, heat and cold, wind and rain encompassed all physical experiences on earth.**

CHI AND YINYANG

Later, *chi* was brought into the system of yinyang so that it now neatly fits in with the whole story of the Dao, yinyang and *chi* all working together to create the universe.

Within yinyang theory there are two types of *chi*: yin *chi* (陰氣), which creates matter, and yang *chi* (陽氣), which animates matter. In a constant state of change and movement, *chi* brings microscopic matter together into a living being and then, when the being's *chi* has been extinguished, the matter returns to its microscopic parts and reforms as something else.

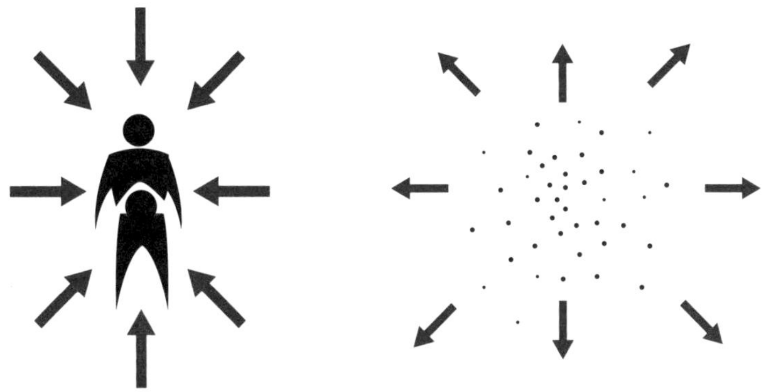

ABOVE: *Chi* comes together when a being comes to life and disperses when that being dies.

This idea of yin and yang *chi* features heavily in Traditional Chinese Medicine. When yang *chi* diminishes, yin *chi* takes its place. When both forms of *chi* leave a living being, the *chi* returns to the source. The constant pulsating in the universe between yin and yang *chi* is what we call life.

YIN AND YANG *CHI*		
IDEOGRAM	CHINESE	JAPANESE
陰氣	*Yin chi*	*In ki*
陽氣	*Yang chi*	*Yo ki*

One key question is just how yinyang and *chi* interact. In its simplest terms, yinyang is the movement and *chi* is the energy associated with that movement, which animates life. The two illustrations overleaf explain this relationship in simple terms.

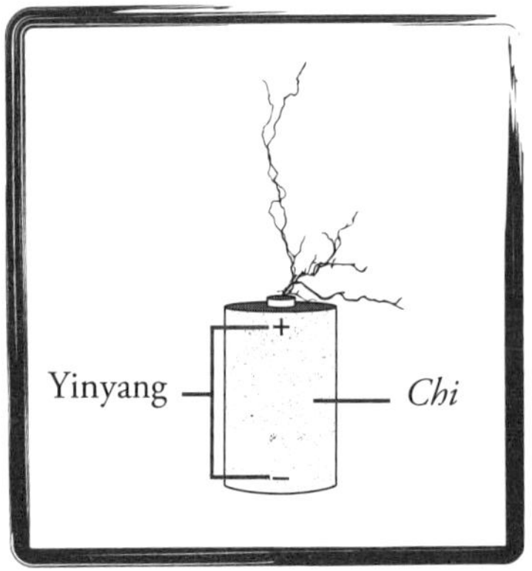

ABOVE: If a battery is the Dao, the positive and negative poles are yin and yang and the potential power inside is *chi*.

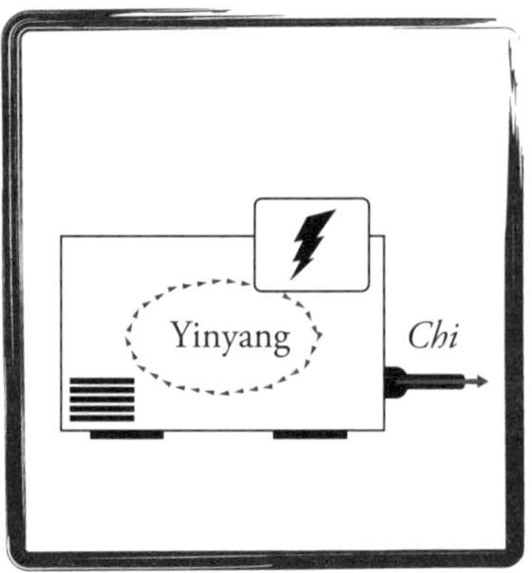

ABOVE: If an electrical generator is the Dao, the movement of the engine in the generator is yinyang and the power output from the generator is *chi*.

Yinyang is the movement and *chi* is the energy. Yin *chi* creates things and yang *chi* gives them their nature and power. Life comes together and then returns to the source in an unending rhythm of forming and dissolving.

WHAT POWERS THE DAO?

If the Dao is a battery or generator, where did the fuel for that battery or generator come from? Basically, this is the same question as, "If God created the universe, what created God?" The Dao and God are eternal. There is nothing before them or beyond them, they are the creators and have never been created. If this is too difficult to accept, consider that the Dao is outside of your universe or understanding and that a power from outside moves this "generator" of the universe, which in turn powers your life. If there was something before the Dao then it is beyond scientific comprehension and you will never understand it. Instead focus on your own existence within the Dao.

THE *CHI* OF HEAVEN AND THE *CHI* OF EARTH

Heaven has its own form of *chi*, as does the earth. The *chi* of heaven descends, the *chi* of earth accumulates. Water evaporates into the sky and rain and snow fall from the heavens. The *chi* of heaven is always intermingling with the *chi* of the earth in the place where humans exist. Therefore, the *chi* of heaven, the *chi* of earth and the *chi* of humans all mix together and affect each other within our own landscape.

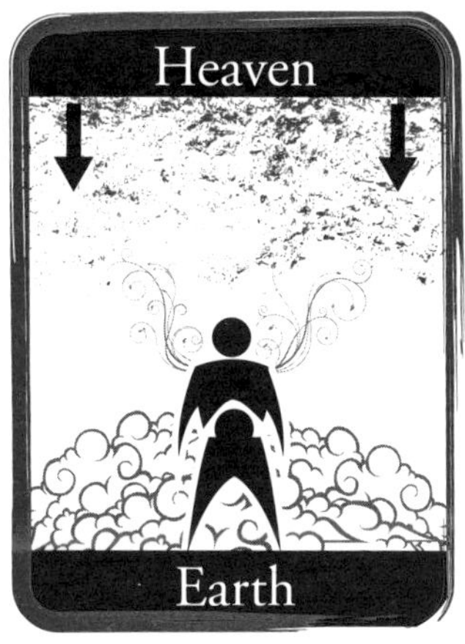

ABOVE: The three aspects of heaven, earth and humans.

Remember, yin *chi* hovers around the earth while yang *chi* descends.

Chi is sometimes associated with wind and human *chi* considered as a "wind" that circulates through a human body. This makes a direct connection between the idea of the *chi* of heaven and the *chi* of humans.

The *chi* of heaven falls and mingles with the *chi* of earth in the realm of humans.

THE FOUR STATES OF *CHI*

Chi can be said to be in four states, positions or situations:

- When *chi* gathers together there is life.
- When there is no *chi* there is no life.
- When *chi* declines or is blocked there is illness.
- When *chi* fully evaporates there is death.

***Chi* is always on the move, but when it is blocked or stagnant there will be illness and when it is used up there will be death. If no *chi* is present in the first place then life does not even begin.**

THE FIVE STAGES OF *CHI*

Now is the time to start relating *chi* to your own being. The concept of the five stages of *chi* will help you to understand the times when your own *chi* is at its strongest and its weakest. Know that you are the product of ever-moving and ever-changing *chi*, that one day your own *chi* will expire and that the parts of your body will disintegrate, but also that you are a part of the fundamental matter of the universe and you will go on after death in another form. You are filled with the energy of the most powerful thing in creation, creation itself.

These five stages of power can be described as follows. Understand that the order of the stages and their translations differ from text to text, so the ideograms have been given here for clarity.

1. 王 – flourishing (very strong)
2. 相 – harmony (strong)
3. 囚 – captured (average strength)
4. 老 – hibernation (weak)
5. 死 – death (very weak)

SEASONAL STRENGTH OF THE FIVE PHASES AND THE FOUR DIRECTIONS

The five stages of *chi* strength are connected to the Five Phases, the four seasons and the four directions. The first table on the opposite page shows how the *chi* of each of the Five Phases rises and falls in strength according to the season.

The second table, based on information from the seventeenth-century samurai scroll the Ippei Yoko, focuses instead on when *chi* associated with each of the four directions is at its strongest. Note that ICP stands for "inter-cardinal points", i.e. northeast, southeast, northwest and southwest. The "transition" column refers to the transitional periods of 18 days between each season in eastern thought. These were made up of the last nine days of one season and the first nine days of the next.

CHI STRENGTH ACCORDING TO SEASON AND PHASE						
IDEOGRAM	STAGE	STRENGTH	SPRING	SUMMER	AUTUMN	WINTER
王	Flourishing	Very strong	Wood	Fire	Metal	Water
相	Harmony	Strong	Fire	Earth	Water	Wood
囚	Captured	Average	Metal	Water	Fire	Earth
老	Hibernation	Weak	Water	Wood	Earth	Metal
死	Death	Very weak	Earth	Metal	Wood	Fire

CHI STRENGTH ACCORDING TO SEASON AND DIRECTION						
STAGE	STRENGTH	SPRING	SUMMER	AUTUMN	WINTER	TRANSITION
Flourishing	Very strong	East	South	West	North	ICP
Harmony	Strong	South	ICP	North	East	West
Captured	Average	West	North	South	ICP	East
Hibernation	Weak	North	East	ICP	West	South
Death	Very weak	ICP	West	East	South	North

Using these two tables together, you can pinpoint the season in which a certain phase and direction are particularly powerful – in order to time your activities to make best use of strong *chi*. This will make more sense when you have read the later chapters, but we will now work through the system using spring as an example.

In spring the east flourishes

East is the strongest direction in spring and the element of wood is at its strongest. Remember, wood is the element for the direction of east and for spring. This combination sees *chi* flourishing at full power.

In spring there is harmony with the south

Wood generates fire in the cycle of generation. This means that because wood is strongest in the east and fire in the south, during spring south is in harmony with the east. South is the direction that supports strength in spring – it is second in strength to the east during this time.

In spring the west is considered as captured

The element of metal destroys wood in the destruction cycle. Therefore, the element of metal and the direction of west (which is the direction of metal) are of only average strength in spring, meaning it is "captured" in the middle level of power.

In the spring the north is in hibernation

The element of water generates wood. Therefore, in spring north (which is the direction of water) generates east (which is the direction of wood), but it is still a weak direction even though it is not in conflict. It is fourth in strength.

In spring the inter-cardinal points are positions of death

Spring is of the wood element, but in spring the inter-cardinal points are of the element of earth. In the cycle of destruction wood is in conflict with earth, which means that in spring the inter-cardinal points are in a phase of "death". These directions have the weakest *chi* in spring.

The other parts of the year can be laid out just as well using this system.

☯ *Chi* fluctuates in strength according to season, direction and phase. Knowing the circumstances when it is at its strongest and weakest is vital for maintaining your own *chi* levels.

VOLUME OR INTENSITY?

Does the amount of chi *in a body decrease and increase, or does the volume stay constant while the power level varies in intensity? Reading the old texts does not give a clear answer to this question. However, the most important thing is to visualize* chi *as a pulsating energy resource that can be abundant or scant depending on the situation. Whether it is a question of volume or power output, the principle of riding the waves of the universe applies just the same.*

WORKING WITH YINYANG:

Build your *chi*

Now you should have a better understanding of what *chi* is and where it is from, how it creates matter and how it animates life. Some people treat *chi* as a magical force, but this is not the best way to view it. First, appreciate that you are alive with *chi*, understand your own position within the landscape and see that all things are connected through a shared energy. Then understand that each season of the year has phases of power and that certain directions are more powerful with *chi* at certain times. For example, in spring you should gather *chi* from the east, but in summer that power will change to the south, and so on. Take actions that will boost your *chi*, whether that is visiting an acupuncturist or simply sitting in the sun for a while if you are feeling drained.

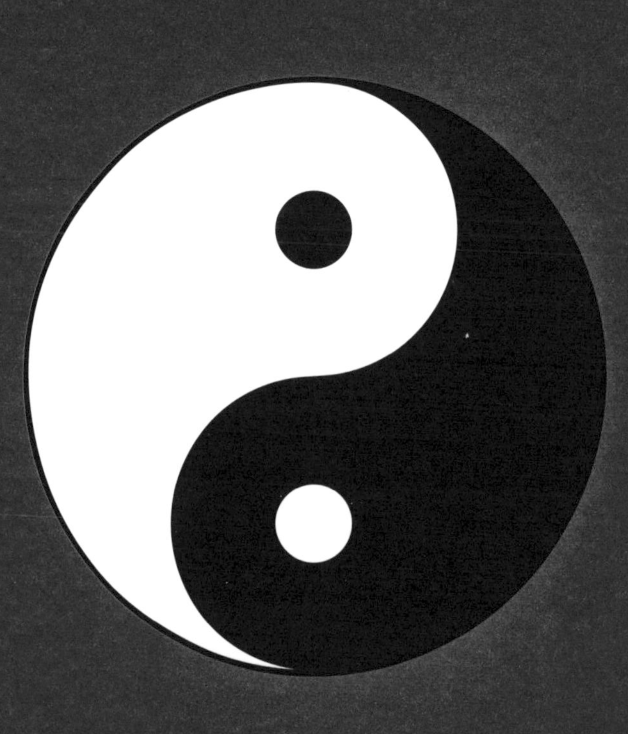

CHAPTER 14

THE WIDER LANDSCAPE

THE WIDER LANDSCAPE

It is now time to take a deeper look at how yinyang affects the world around you on a more personal level, how the places that surround you are defined by the concept of yinyang. Here we will see how the concept of time is fundamental to understanding human experience and discover how divination and *feng shui* were developed to help humans engage more with the natural world.

TIMING

The Chinese ideogram for time is *shi* (時), meaning "seasons", and yinyang takes a seasonal view of timing. To have correct timing in yinyang is to understand when to do something within the year. For example, it is hard to start a fire during a storm or collect water during a drought.

The principle of correct timing applies not only to interactions with the natural world but also to those with other humans. Do not talk loudly in a quiet train carriage, but do not talk quietly at a loud festival. Do not see timing in terms of hours and minutes; instead see it as the correct combination of action and situation.

☯ **Timing means choosing actions that are appropriate to the situation.**

DAYS, MONTHS AND YEARS

The Chinese have the same word for day as for sun (日) because in one day the sun rises and sets. Likewise, the Chinese word for month is moon (月) because they used the moon to count their months. The word for year (年) originated from the ideogram for rice grains because a year equates to a single crop cycle. Day (yang) turns to night (yin), summer (yang) turns to winter (yin) and thus the cycle of yinyang rotates on the same axis as the wheel of the year.

NATURAL DISASTERS

Natural disasters are the result of an extreme movement from yin to yang or yang to yin. They can sometimes be anticipated by observing deviations from the natural order, such as unexpected weather changes or earth tremors, which indicate that an imbalance has built up. Such imbalances in yinyang do not mean that the earth itself is out of balance, but they can be the precursor to a sudden corrective movement in yinyang that is dangerous or uncomfortable for humans.

Note that these sudden changes are more likely to happen in so-called disaster hotspots like flood plains and earthquake fault lines. Yinyang theory tells us that we should put ourselves in a place where yinyang serves us well, so to live in a high-risk zone is against this teaching.

☯ **Natural disasters can be anticipated by careful observation of the landscape, but to live in a location at high risk of such events is against the teachings of yinyang.**

THE SOLSTICE AND THE EQUINOX

The summer solstice is the longest day of the year and it is often celebrated as such. Remember, however, that this occasion also marks the beginning of a decline in day length. While representing the highest expression of yang within the year, this day is also when yin is born. The reverse is true of the winter solstice. The shortest, darkest day of the year and the height of yin, it also marks the birth of yang when light starts to enter the world again. Equinoxes, which are the two days of the year when day and night are of equal length, represent a perfect balance of yin and yang.

☯ **The solstices are the points when either yin or yang is at its strongest and its counterpart is at its weakest, whereas at the equinoxes yin and yang are perfectly balanced.**

THE FOUR SEASONS

From the depths of winter to the very height of summer, the seasons gradually change from yin to yang and back again in a never-ending cycle. Spring and summer are yang; autumn and winter are yin. However, there are two ways of defining the relationship between each pair of seasons in terms of yinyang. One system is based on growth and the other is based on power. At first they seem contradictory, but they are just based on two different but complementary aspects of yinyang.

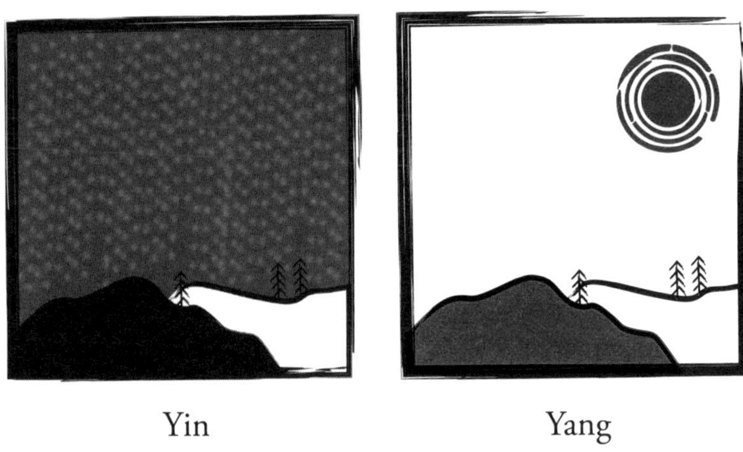

Yin Yang

ABOVE: Winter is yin, summer is yang.

The table below summarizes the two systems.

SEASON	YINYANG BASED ON GROWTH	YINYANG BASED ON POWER
Spring	Yang in a phase of yang (because it is growing toward summer)	Yang in a phase of yin (because it is the less powerful yang season)
Summer	Yang in a phase of yin (because it is declining toward autumn)	Yang in a phase of yang (because it is the more powerful yang season)

SEASON	YINYANG BASED ON GROWTH	YINYANG BASED ON POWER
Autumn	Yin in a phase of yang (because it is growing toward winter)	Yin in a phase of yin (because it is the less powerful yin season)
Winter	Yin in a phase of yin (because it is declining toward spring)	Yin in a phase of yang (because it is the more powerful yin season)

Taking spring as an example, you can see it as the yang portion of the yang half of the year because it is the period when the amount of yang is growing each day in the approach to the summer solstice. Alternatively, you might say that it is the yin portion of the yang half of the year because yang is less powerful during spring than it is during summer.

The first relationship is about birth and death, a movement from yin to yang; the second relationship is about high and low power. This is a good example of how yin and yang should only be seen in relation to each other and not as fixed labels.

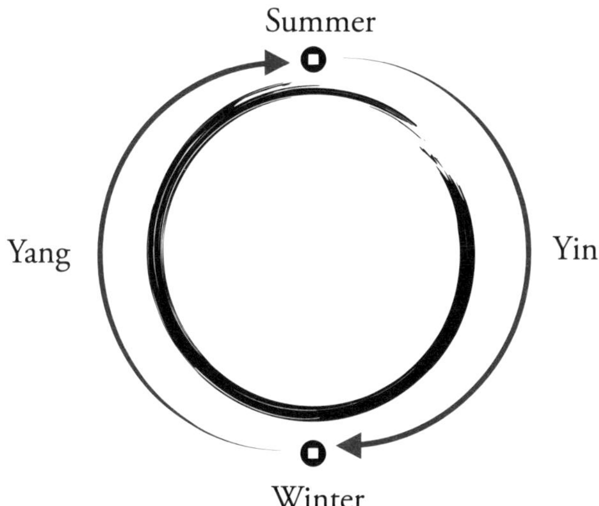

ABOVE: Yin and yang move through the seasons in a constant cycle of change.

SEASONS, EMOTIONS AND CLIMATE

The seasons are associated not only with certain types of climate but also with certain emotions. However, it is important to be aware that there are multiple systems of emotion in Asian thought, and it is easy to get them mixed up if you are not careful. One such system, shown in the table below, is connected to yinyang and Chinese thought, while others are based on the teachings of Buddhism.

All systems discuss how the mind can change quickly from one emotion to another and there are different theories as to which emotions change into which depending on the school of thought. Simply understand that emotions in Asian thought have multiple meanings and that some of them are related to the seasons. For example, spring is associated with joy and anger but these are only base emotions for that season. The mind can change quickly.

SEASONS, CLIMATE AND EMOTIONS		
SEASON	CLIMATE	EMOTION
Spring	Warmth / Wind	Joy / Anger
Summer	Heat / The sun	Happiness / Contentment
Autumn	Coolness / Dryness	Wrath / Unhappiness
Winter	Cold / The moon	Mourning / Fear

☯ **Spring and summer are yang; autumn and winter are yin. In terms of growth, spring and autumn are yang compared to summer and winter, but yin in terms of power. Each season can be associated with certain weather conditions and emotions.**

RIVERS

Although water itself is a yin element, different aspects of a river such as its source, the direction it flows and its shallow and deep areas are divided into yin and yang.

- The source of a river is an element of yin.
- The place it flows to is an element of yang.
- The darker and deeper parts of the river are the element of yin.
- The clearer and shallower parts are the element of yang.

A river flows from yin to yang. It has yin depths and yang shallows.

TIDES

Most of the time when something is at full power it is considered to be yang, and when it is at low power it is yin. However, the opposite is the case with tides. Water is of yin, so the more of it there is, the more yin energy there is. When a tide is in, it is at its most powerful and is full of yin energy. When the tide ebbs away and there is less water, yin energy drops and yang energy increases.

When the tide is high the power of yin is high, when the tide is low the power of yin is low.

THE TIDES AND DEATH

There is believed to be a connection between the tides and the day of the month a person is likely to die. This is known in Japanese as chishigo.

CHANGING THE WEATHER

According to yinyang theory, humans can help change the weather in the following ways.

IF IT IS TOO HOT AND DRY

Heat and dryness are yang forms of energy that in excess can bring drought and devastate crops. Therefore, if there is too much yang energy in the world, people need to increase the yin energy to counter it. They can do this by closing the south gate of the city (south is yang) to stop yang energy flowing into the area. Men (yang) should stay hidden indoors, while women (yin) should go out and take an active role in public. Sex between a man and a woman purges yang energy and builds up yin energy, so heterosexual couples should have much more sex. Finally, all men should spend their time making women happy so that the population shines with yin brightness.

IF IT IS TOO COLD AND WET

Cold and wetness are yin forms of energy that can flood and freeze places, bringing misery to all. To reduce an excess of yin energy, women should stay indoors while men should go about in public. Historically, families would even send their female members away to unaffected regions during times of flood or extreme cold in order to increase yang *chi*. The men would drum on the ground to bring about a movement from yin to yang. Men and women should not have sex during these times.

☯ **Drought is caused by an excess of yang and floods come from an excess of yin. Men and women can restore the balance by engaging in or refraining from certain activities.**

FENG SHUI

"First is your destiny, second is luck and third is feng shui.*"*

Ancient Chinese saying

Literally translated as "wind-water", *feng shui* is the practice of positioning yourself within nature in accordance with yinyang theory so as to gather the *chi* of the world, promote proper flow and generate prosperity and good health. It involves mastering three main aspects:

- **the timing of heaven** – changing seasons and weather
- **the benefits of earth** – natural resources and the bounty of the land
- **the waxing and waning of yin and yang**

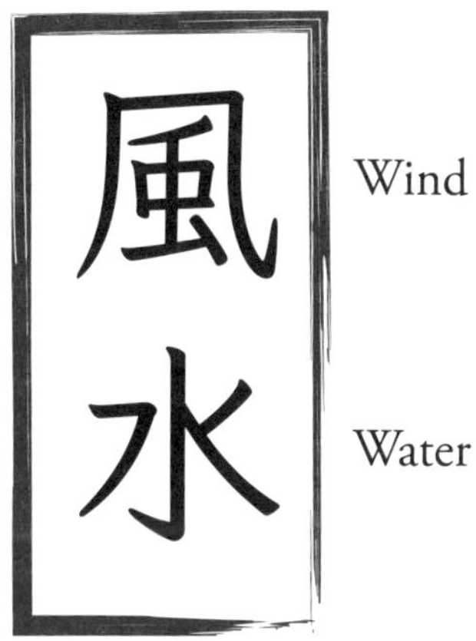

ABOVE: The ideograms for *feng shui.*

Feng shui was originally developed to help in the planning of funerary rites and the placement of tombs for the dead, which were known as "houses of yin". This was done so that the spirit aspect known as *po* (see chapter 18) had a proper place to reside, and it was also a way for humans to understand their position in the cosmos.

Later, *feng shui* developed into a set of complex architectural rules and detailed teachings on placement, an overview of which is given below. These are just the basic aspects of the practice and each location will present different challenges. All kinds of factors, such as colour, road positions and the shapes of neighbouring buildings, need to be taken into account. Therefore, to be sure of benefiting from *feng shui* you will either need to become a master of the art or bring one in for advice. However, be aware that it is a belief system, so be careful who you employ.

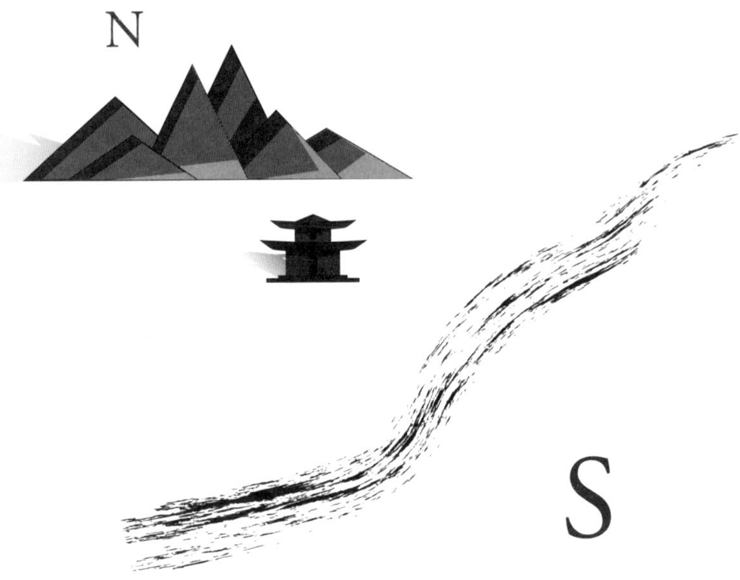

ABOVE: A well-positioned house: facing the sun with hills behind it and water to the front.

FACE THE SUN

According to *feng shui* the front of your house should face the south (or the north if you are in the southern hemisphere). This means that the sun will rise in full view and keep your house in sunlight for the longest possible time and the land around the house will be good for growing crops.

USE WATER TO COLLECT *CHI*

When *chi* hits water it slows down and gathers. Therefore, you can use water to stop *chi* from escaping, keeping your position well supplied with energy.

HAVE WATER TO THE FRONT

There should be water to the front of your sun-facing house so that in the hot summer any warm winds that come from that direction will be cooled by the water. The water does not have to be very close to the house, and it goes without saying that you should not build on a flood plain.

WATER MUST NOT SCATTER

Water that falls down from a height and scatters is considered to be bad. Water must either collect or flow in a steady stream. Otherwise, the *chi* held by the water will disperse into the air and the wind will take it away.

AVOID WINDY PLACES

Wind will blow *chi* away from your location, leaving it barren.

HAVE MOUNTAINS TO THE BACK

If your house or position faces the sun, as it ideally should, there should not be mountains in front, because these will cast a shadow over you. However, it is good to have mountains to the rear. They create a barrier that traps beneficial *chi* near and around your home and also shelter you from cold northern winds.

BENEFIT FROM BRIDGES

A nearby water bridge can be a great asset. Bridges lock the *chi* gathered by the water into position, making them places of high energy.

PINPOINT DIRECTIONS AND POSITIONS OF IMPORTANCE

In Asia, the place where a person sits has great significance and in the past rooms were set up around the position or seat of honour. The hierarchy of positions in the east, from highest honour to lowest, are:

1. central seat facing south
2. side seat facing east or west
3. seat close to the outside of the building facing north

Note that a "central" seat is generally not in the centre of a room. More often than not, it will be on an internal wall in a room. However, it is central in terms of the building as a whole. Also, take note of the position of the sun in this system: the highest-ranking people face the sun; the middle-ranking people have the sun on the side of their face; and the lowest-ranking people have the sun at their back and their faces in shadow. If there needs to be a further delineation within the middle ranks on the sides, then east/left (yang) is higher than west/right (yin).

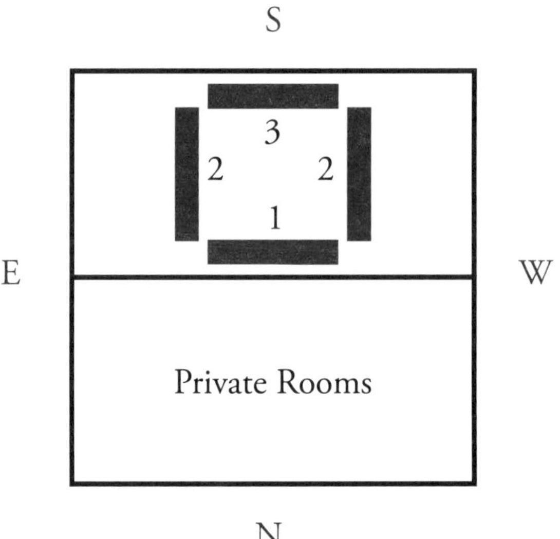

ABOVE: The hierarchy of seating positions, with the highest-ranking position (1) in the centre of the building and facing south.

FIND AUSPICIOUS DAYS AND TIMES

Feng shui can be used for placement in time as well as space. There are auspicious times to get married, start ventures, change ideas, and so on. The calculation is quite complex, as many factors have to be taken into account. However, be aware that there are certain days on which things should be done and other days on which they should not be done.

FIVE SYSTEMS INTO ONE

Feng shui brings together the following five systems into one overarching system:

- Yinyang
- The Five Phases
- The 10 Heavenly Stems
- The 12 Earthly Branches
- The 12 Blessings and Curses (see chapter 20)

When the complex relationships between these five systems are understood, *feng shui* starts to take shape.

☯ *Feng shui* involves knowing where to be and how to use the weather, and understanding when yin and yang are in power.

THE SEED OF DESTINY

The benefits gained by applying *feng shui* and those allocated by heaven (destiny) are not the same. The best way to fully understand this idea is to consider the life of a seed. A seed is already programmed to become a particular type of plant. That is its destiny and nothing can change it. However, the positioning of the seed – the type of soil it is in and the amount of water and sun it receives – will affect how it grows. Furthermore, if you train the plant, prune it and feed it correctly, it will grow much better than one that has been neglected. This is the idea of destiny combined with *feng shui* (human positioning).

☯ Some aspects of our existence are preordained; others can be changed for the better through self-cultivation.

WORKING WITH YINYANG:
Follow the principles of *feng shui*

Understand that your position within the greater and lesser landscape is a core aspect of yinyang theory. Use your observation of the seasons and the landscape as your clock. True time is not defined by minutes, hours and days so much as by natural movements. Stumbling out of the rhythm of yinyang can lead you into adversity. However, by correct positioning within the landscape using the principles of *feng shui*, your home and whole life can be a source of powerful, vibrant energy.

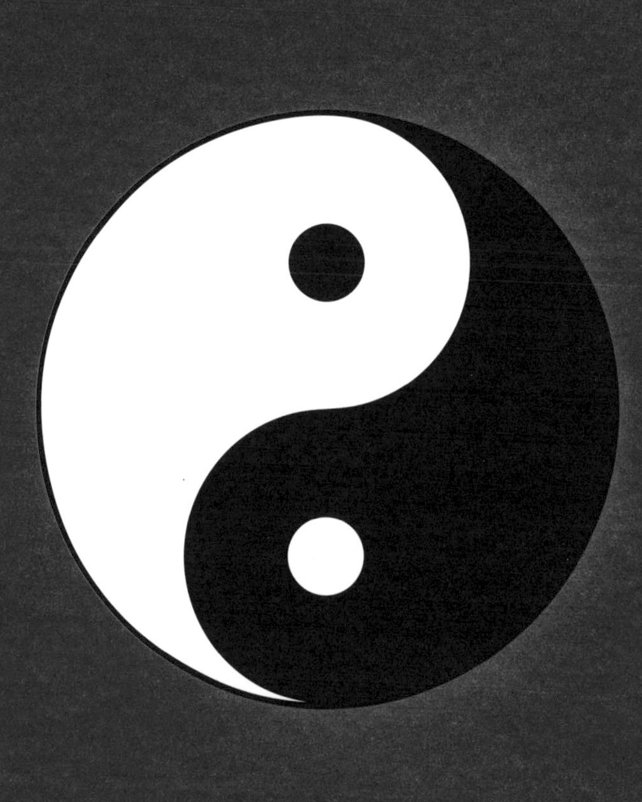

CHAPTER 15

YOUR RELATIONSHIP TO THE UNIVERSE

YOUR RELATIONSHIP TO THE UNIVERSE

You have now positioned yourself within the landscape and understood it as a creation and manifestation of the Dao and the movement of yinyang with the animating power of *chi*, and you have seen that there are directions and times when *chi* is at its strongest. Now it is time to delve deeper into the relationships that form within the universe, so that you can better appreciate the world from your own point of view as you observe the majesty of creation around you.

HUMAN INTERFERENCE

Human behaviour can create an imbalance in the natural order of yinyang, leading to a build-up of either yin or yang. In the past, Daoist masters would take care to ensure that the community was acting in harmony with the will of heaven and watch for portents of impending doom if it was not behaving correctly. If a whole nation is in such a state of incorrectness, then heaven's response to this imbalance can be on the level of a major earthquake, flood or other natural disaster with a high fatality rate.

☯ If one person is acting in a way that throws yinyang out of balance, only they will be affected; if all people do so, it will affect the whole world.

HEAVEN, EARTH AND HUMANS

One of the central themes in Chinese thought is the relationship between heaven, earth and humans. The link is yinyang, which moves between heaven and earth, affects the landscape and can be interacted with by humans.

A good example of this relationship is the planting of crops. Humans plant crops in the earth, but it takes heaven to nourish them so that they grow. Humans harvest them and the waste degrades and replenishes the earth.

All three are needed for proper human existence.

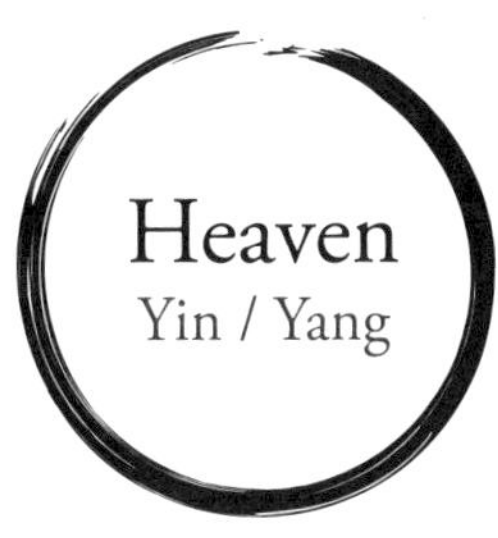

While heaven cannot be altered, the land should be properly cultivated and humans should aspire for perfection both within themselves and within the landscape. There are three basic levels of humans classified according to the level of perfection they have achieved. These are:

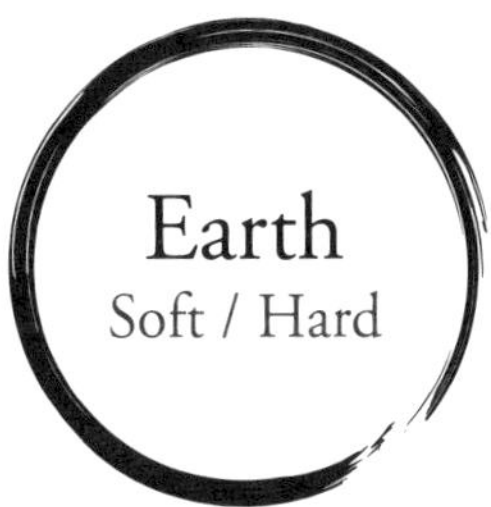

1. Standard person (instinctual)
2. Superior person (cultivated and refined)
3. Sage (in harmony with heaven and the Way)

A standard person is someone who acts on instinct, lives life without progress but is content with the status quo. A superior person is one who follows the correct patterns of social behaviour and who is educated and stands out from the standard people. A sage has moved beyond refinement and understands all the different aspects of yinyang and can fully comprehend how nature works in relation to their life. A sage is able to profit from correct harmony with yinyang, live in peace with others and enrich the earth, maintaining a correct relationship with the universe.

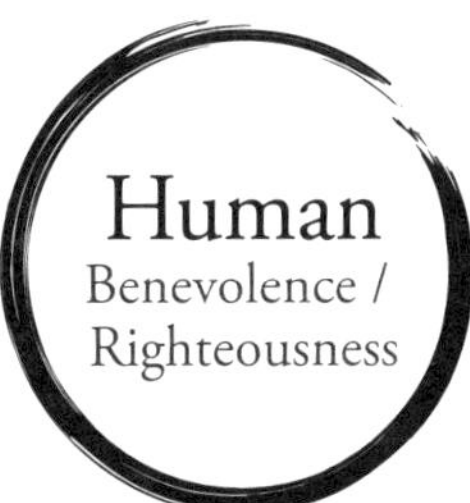

ABOVE: Heaven, earth and humans and their associations.

Ritual and community events are a way for humans to strengthen their relationship with the landscape and heaven. Traditional events and gatherings bring harmony to the people and the world, allowing yinyang to flow in the correct way, with music and dance both representing and actualizing this harmony.

☯ **Heaven, earth and humans are inextricably linked by yinyang. Humans can strengthen this link by living in harmony with yinyang.**

THE RELATIONSHIP BETWEEN YIN AND YANG

The relationship between yin and yang can be described in four different ways:

- *Yin and yang as direct opposites of each other: they are at opposite ends of a spectrum.*
- *Yin and yang as completely independent of each other: they are separate entities with their own identities. For example, the sun simply stands as yang and water stands as yin and they are not viewed in relation to each other.*
- *Yin and yang consuming each other: yang energy can devour yin energy and vice versa.*
- *Yin and yang transforming into each other: day becomes night, night becomes day, heat becomes cold, cold becomes heat. This idea of yin and yang giving way to each other in an endless cycle of change is known as* zhuanhua *(*轉化*).*

HEAVEN, EARTH AND TIME

There is heaven, there is earth and there is time. Heaven is concerned with time and season. Earth presents location and position. It is the task of the human to understand these factors and put themselves in the most beneficial position at the right time to do a given activity so that they can gain the most from yinyang.

The Chinese term *yinyang fenbu* (陰陽分布) means to look at a geographical location and identify where yin and yang will fall in relation to the sun. It involves asking yourself these questions:

- Is it the correct time to do this activity?
- Is the location correct?
- Does this location offer what I need?

For example, when positioning a garden, building a house, identifying a picnic spot, it is always best to understand where south is and track where the sun will rise and set and how the shadows move over the land each day. This way you will not position yourself in shadow or on the wrong side of a hill but will find a comfortable spot either for a temporary setting or a permanent establishment. Always remember your own relationship to the environment and think of the cycles of life around you so that you do not put effort into being in the wrong place at the wrong time doing the wrong thing.

To be in the correct position at the correct time doing the correct thing will bring you in harmony with the movement of yinyang.

Yinyang =

correct resources
correct situation
correct timing

= success

ABOVE: The formula for harmony with yinyang.

THE CONCEPT OF GENERATION

Your position within the universe is not static, and you have to move with the waves of change. All things go through periods of generation (生), which can take the form of either transformation or reproduction.

TRANSFORMATION

Examples of transformation include one season becoming the next, water evaporating into the air and becoming a cloud then condensing into rain, and cliffs becoming rocks, rocks becoming pebbles and pebbles becoming sand.

REPRODUCTION

Most living creatures go through life and death and have to reproduce to continue the existence of their species. Acorns become trees, babies are born, the old die, generation after generation move in and out of life and death.

Yinyang can never be made to stand still. Substances transform into new substances or states, living beings reproduce to continue their species.

ALL THINGS HAVE PHASES

Another way to see your relationship to the world was put forward by the ancient Chinese:

- Heaven has seasons.
- Earth has natural territories and boundaries.
- All things have phases.

The term "things" here is from the concept of "ten thousand things", meaning that all of creation goes through phases. We exist within the boundaries of the earth and gravity, the seasons move across the land with us, but we, like all other objects of creation, go through phases. In this sense, we are no different from a wooden chair, which is made, used, becomes dilapidated and has a final demise into firewood and ash. Birth, flourishing, decline, death and dissolution. You have to come to terms with your own eventual death and dissolution, but in the knowledge that you will return to the Great Ultimate and always be part of a changing universe.

☯ **All of creation goes through phases, from birth to dissolution.**

HEAVEN IS BEYOND HUMAN KNOWLEDGE

Heaven contains yin and yang but it also contains time. Without time, yin and yang would have no room to change and mutate between each other. Earth has distance; it contains places that are near or far, broad or narrow. Some of these places give life, others kill. Heaven has no distance. For the ancient Chinese, it was an intangible place beyond the earth where they could never go. So from the Dao comes the flow of yin and yang and the movement of time; on earth there are perceptible aspects, such as distance, depth and height, but also danger and sustenance.

☯ **A human looks up to heaven to see the weather and the passage of time. On earth the seasons roll around and humans flow in and out of relationships, but they can never see beyond the stars.**

COMMUNICATING WITH HEAVEN

Humans have always striven to communicate with the "entity" or power behind creation. For the ancient Chinese, that power was the Dao and their means of communication with the Dao was correct interaction with yinyang. Correctly identifying yinyang and working in harmony with it and riding on its currents will produce a positive relationship with the Dao, which will lead to a healthy, fruitful and meaningful life. This is your relationship with the Dao and it involves no one but you and the Dao.

☯ **Heaven sees all and all will be accounted for in the end.**

ACHIEVING HARMONY

Harmony (和) is all things working in unison to create a perfect whole. There are two ways in which it can be understood: as constructed harmony and as blended harmony.

CONSTRUCTED HARMONY

Constructed harmony involves individual parts cooperating with each other to create a desired effect. An orchestra is made up of separate parts. Violinists and percussionists can be picked out as being distinct from each other, but when they are combined they can create a dramatic performance. Afterwards, the parts can be separated again and harmony becomes disorder. It is only the temporary coming together of the individual parts that creates a perfect relationship.

BLENDED HARMONY

In blended harmony the individual parts are changed by the process of blending into a perfect whole. Once combined, they cannot be separated. For example, the eggs, flour, butter and sugar that come together to make a cake cannot be identified or extracted once the cake has been mixed and baked. Similarly, pigments for paints are mixed with oils and combined on a canvas to create harmony in the form of a great work of art.

THE WRONG MIX

Harmony relies on the right combination of components or ingredients.

A klaxon going off in the middle of a symphony causes disharmony, and too much salt in a dish will throw off the balance of flavours. It is the same when you are interacting with yinyang on earth to create a harmonious relationship with heaven. Too much yin or yang at the wrong time will disrupt any form of accord you have with heaven. Always do what feels correct, not what you think is correct.

☯ **The world is a form of constructed harmony, but yin and yang blend together and flow within it.**

AS ABOVE, SO BELOW

Many Daoist traditions teach that understanding the heavens can be a key to understanding the earth. What is in the stars represents things that will happen in the world and will affect the lives of humans. This involves looking for omens and portents and reading various aspects of the night sky. If heaven is the macrocosm, earth is the microcosm and heaven controls earth.

☯ **The world and the heavens are connected and humans can change both their own environment and the heavens by performing actions that emit a certain *chi*.**

THE GREAT PLAN

As the theory of the universe and its connection to humans became more complex in Chinese thought, a nine-level system was set out known as the Great Plan. This consists of:

1. The Five Phases
2. The five human behaviours
3. The eight parts of government
4. The five regulations of time

5. The central power of government
6. The three virtues
7. The investigation of anything appearing doubtful
8. The understanding of omens and portents
9. Taking heed of the five delights and the six calamities

It is believed that if all people investigate and follow all aspects of the Great Plan, then peace and prosperity will reign over society and heaven will bestow great rewards on the people.

For the world to be correct, all humans have to understand the universe's plan.

HEAVEN RESPONDS TO HUMANS

Heaven will respond to humans depending on their actions. Therefore, pure and good people have a good connection to heaven, while evil people have a poor connection to the benefits of heaven (though they may still be rich in material benefits such as money). There are three aspects to this relationship:

- the correct effort at the correct time and place
- consideration for the future and the best actions to prepare for it
- taking responsibility for your own actions

People often mistake money for a reward, but having too much money is the same as having too little. Both make us uncomfortable – either physically or emotionally, or both. When you have achieved the correct relationship with heaven by your actions you will be rewarded with comfort, not riches.

Heaven wants to give you what you need, but first you must learn the best way to behave and position yourself.

HUMANS ARE NOT CONTROLLED BY THE DAO

It is crucial to understand that we are free to react in any way we wish to any situation. Treat all situations as heaven presenting us with an opportunity to do the right thing. If we are not following the Way, we are making the wrong choices. Our aim must be to align ourselves with correct action so that we can progress within the world and maintain our position within the embracing flow of the Dao.

Humans are produced by the Dao, but they are not controlled by the Dao.

THE MORALITY OF THE DAO

It is said that the Dao is neither good nor bad, that it has no morality in itself. However, it is also said that the Dao continually presents humans with opportunities to act correctly and that it rewards right behaviour and punishes wrong behaviour. One could argue that this demonstrates an indirect form of morality – a point countered by some schools of thought, which say that human action leaves no impression on the Dao.

What, then, is the purpose of our existence? When we die we return to the Dao to enter a state of "non-being" or more correctly a state of potential. In theory what happens next is that our "essence" is put back into creation, most likely in another form to experience the world again. There are many avenues to this debate, but they all take us back to the idea that the Dao is unknowable and that we can only guess at its intentions.

The Dao is neither good nor bad, but gives us the opportunity to be good or bad. It is up to us to find the right path and follow it.

WORKING WITH YINYANG:
Try to understand the universe's plan

Having a clear fix of yourself within the universe and the landscape, observing heaven and earth and understanding creation, you have the pulse of yinyang. Know that life and death are flowing around you at all times, that a complex set of relationships governs the dynamic state of the world, and that the world is not always a safe, comfortable place. It is your task to identify these waves and patterns, to learn how the world works and how heaven wants you to act. You have to form a relationship with the universe. Take what you need without taking too much. Go out in yang when yang is needed, and retreat to yin when yin is needed. Take responsibility for your own actions and try to make the correct effort at the correct time and place. Learn the best way to behave and position yourself, so that heaven will give you what you need.

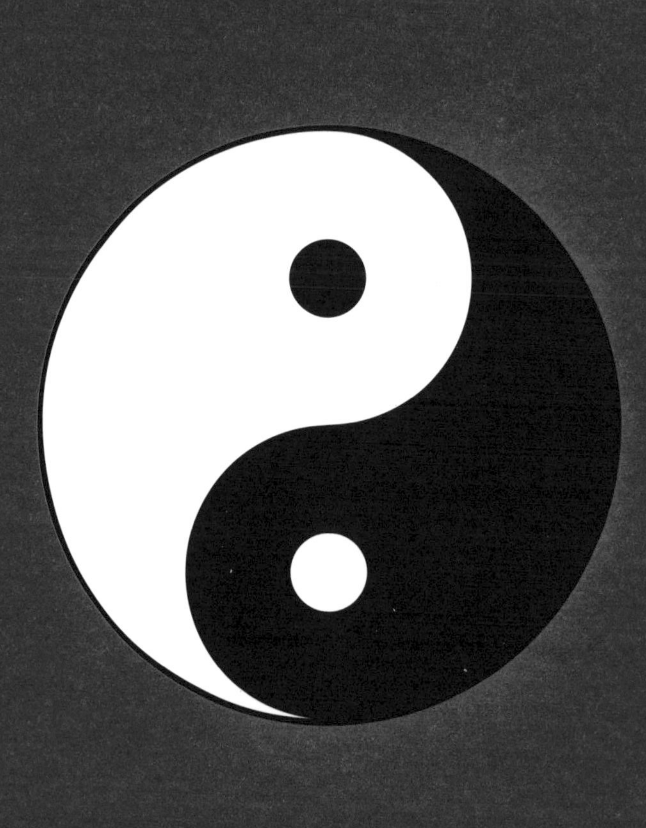

CHAPTER 16

THE FIVE PHASES

THE FIVE PHASES

A question we have not tackled yet is how creation took the leap from the abstract, intangible yin and yang and *chi* to the concrete, physical reality of the world. In order to answer this question we will need to understand the role of the Five Phases, which are states of energy that bridge the gap from source to end product. Every part of the known universe that has physical reality is a vibration of energy at a specific wavelength. Although there are countless mixtures of energy required to make the "ten thousand things" of creation, they can all be broken down into the five basic parts described in this chapter.

WHAT ARE THE FIVE PHASES?

The Five Phases or Elements – fire, metal, water and wood with earth – are five separate states of energy that interact in a cycle together. Although they are named after physical, observable elements, they are not themselves physical. The names are just symbolic representations of different kinds of *chi*. They are always moving, no matter how slowly, and each one takes its turn to be the most prominent. Sometimes they work against each other, sometimes they work with each other, and sometimes they control each other. These five basic parts are very important in Asian thinking and are closely connected to yinyang.

Very early Chinese thought drew a distinction between four elements – fire, metal, water and wood – and earth, which was the place at the centre where the elements existed. At first, fire and water were prominent, but later wood and metal were added. The wood element was understood either as all vegetation, including trees, or sometimes as a wooden plough, which was a traditional implement for churning earth before the metal plough was invented.

It was only later that the idea of relationships and movement between these aspects developed into the complex system we know today. The development was not linear and logical; traditions and variations from different schools were amalgamated over centuries into a standardized teaching.

The Five Phases are states of energy that interact with each other in a number of different cycles. Together they constitute the building blocks of the universe.

PHASES OR ELEMENTS?

Whenever you engage with east Asian systems of thought such as Traditional Chinese Medicine, martial arts and samurai military ways, you will often hear terms such as "five elements", "five aspects" and "five phases". The ancient master Tsou Yen (c.305–240 BC), who was believed to have been the first to link the concept to yinyang, called them the "five powers" and used different ideograms. However, be clear that these are all referring to the same thing.

The most common translation is "five elements", but in this book the concept is referred to as that of the "five phases" in order to underline the idea of movement and transition. While they are indeed five individual elements, each representing a certain type of energy, the most important thing to understand about them is that they move and form relationships with each other.

THE INDIAN AND GREEK ELEMENTS

When reading various books about ancient wisdom you will come across three different lists of elements and their associated systems. These are the Greek, Indian and Chinese elements. Sometimes they appear in the same book without any explanation as to which is which or why they do not match up with each other.

One unproven theory is that the Greek idea of the elements predated and influenced the Indian and Chinese versions. It is suggested that they might have come to Asia as trade routes opened up in ancient times.

In this book we are, of course, dealing with the Chinese elements, but to avoid confusion between the three different systems the Greek and Indian elements are shown below.

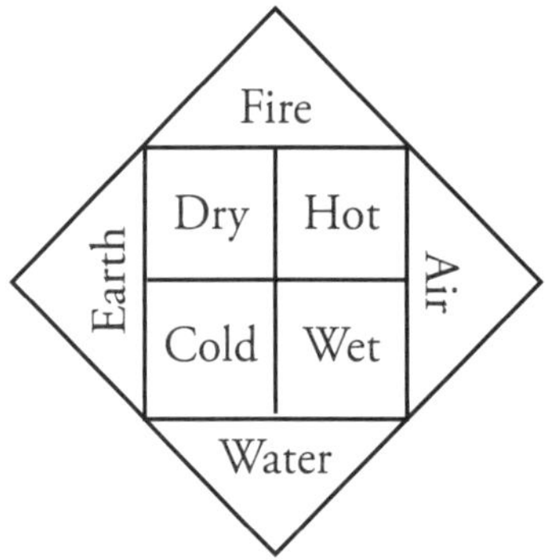

ABOVE: The four Greek elements: fire, air, water and earth.

1	Earth	地
2	Fire	火
3	Sky	空
4	Water	水
5	Wind	風

ABOVE: The five Indian elements: earth, fire, sky, water and wind

The ancient Chinese, Greek and Indian elements are three separate systems. They may have a shared heritage, but it is important not to get them confused.

FIRE AND WATER: A VERTICAL RELATIONSHIP

Early Chinese thought focused on the staples of life: fire and water. Fire licks upward and water trickles downward. Fire is of the element of yang and water is of yin. Together fire and water represent the world in a vertical relationship: a great bonfire burns high up into the sky in the centre of a settlement giving warmth to the tribe and water runs off the surrounding hills to irrigate the crops.

Fire and water also had symbolic significance, as the heat of the sun and the cold dampness of the earth.

Fire and water are the staples of life.

A PHYSICAL AND MENTAL MOVEMENT

The Chinese term we have translated as the Five Phases consists of two ideograms: *wu* (五), which means "five", and *xing* (行), which, broadly speaking, means "movement". However, this second ideogram can mean movement in either a physical or a psychological sense.

Therefore, *wuxing* (五行) can be seen as five movements or behaviours of the mind that can change into each other. From this evolved the concept of *wude* (五德) – five virtues or attitudes that were considered as gifts from heaven to humans. This takes us even further from the physical elements of wood, fire, water and so on into the realm of human behaviour.

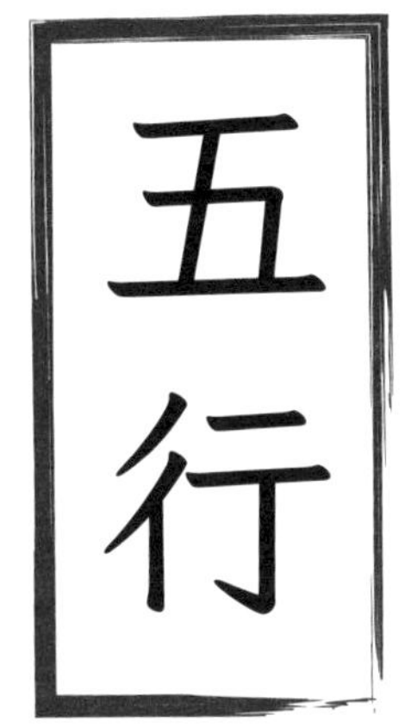

ABOVE: The ideograms comprising *wuxing*, the "Five Phases" (*gogyo* in Japanese).

The movement of the Five Phases takes place not only in the natural world but also within the human mind.

PROBLEMS OF TRANSLATION

For an English speaker, the main barrier to understanding the Five Phases is a linguistic one. English terms such as "element", "phase", "movement", "cycle of creation", "cycle of destruction" and "cycle of control" all have connotations that do not exist in Chinese and so they should be considered only as approximations. For example, different translators refer to one element "controlling", "penetrating" or "destroying" another. Each of these different translations of the same ideogram changes the feeling of how the system works. Be aware of the way different translations can guide you toward different conclusions.

Just because a word has certain connotations in one language, that does not mean it holds the same connotations in another language.

COMPLEMENTARY TEACHINGS

Here would be a good point to pause and explain the difference between the Five Phases and two other teachings. The following three are all different but can be confused with each other when translated.

- ***wuxing* (五行)** – the Five Phases or movements
- ***wucai* (五材)** – the five materials
- ***sancai* (三才)** – the three elements of heaven, earth and humans

The ideogram *cai* (材) found in *wucai* is made up of a "tree" and "natural property", meaning the natural property of an item. Therefore, *wucai* means the five natural properties of the world. Some ancient texts include grain as an extra element and call the system *liu fu* (六府), the "six natural resources".

The term *sancai*, which has a variant of the *cai* ideogram (才), conveys the idea of the three divisions of properties in the universe: within heaven, earth and those beings that live between the two.

☯ **There are three realms (*sancai*): heaven, earth and humans; there are five basic properties of the world (*wucai*); and there are five interrelated forms of energy that pulse within the universe to keep it alive (*wuxing*).**

THE FIVE PHASES: FUNDAMENTAL PROPERTIES AND DIRECTIONS

The following is an overview of the basic characteristics and associated directions of the Five Phases. Remember that their names are only intended to represent the type of energy that they each manifest within the universe or the human body.

The order in which the Five Phases are listed varies, but water often comes first because it is the source of all things and also represents yin. All life must start in yin before it flourishes into yang.

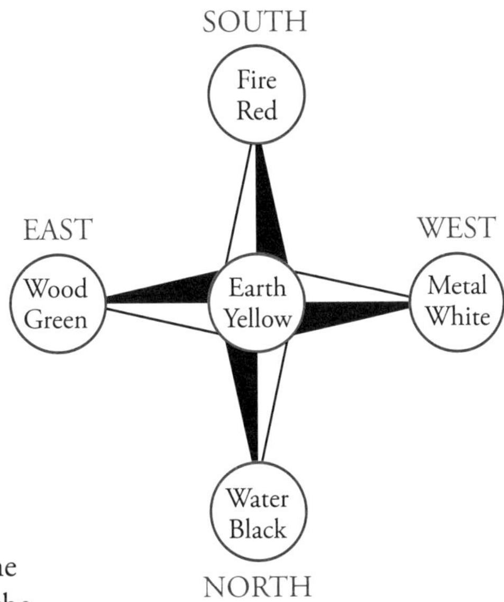

ABOVE: The Five Phases and their associated directions and colours. South is at the top, a common feature on many old Asian maps.

WATER

Water flows from high to low and has the property of coolness. The weather in the north is cold, and therefore water is the element of the north. Water is behind you when you face the sun in the south.

FIRE

Fire flares up, it rises from below and reaches upward. Things that are warm or hot are related to fire. The weather in the south is hot and therefore fire is the element of the south. Fire is to the front when you face the sun as it passes overhead.

WOOD

Wood grows straight up and spreads freely, it flourishes and maintains harmony. The sun rises in the east and the rising of the sun guides the upward growth of branches. Therefore, wood is the element of the east and all things of wood grow up toward the sun. Wood is on the left because it is to the east when you face the sun in the south.

METAL

Metal causes transformation. The sun sets in the west and descends below the horizon and so metal is the element of the west. Metal is on the right because it is to the west when you face the sun in the south.

EARTH

As the giver of life to all things, earth is found at the centre. When you face the sun in the south and you have east and west to your left and right and north to your rear, the earth is directly below your feet.

☯ Cooling water is north, burning fire is south, upward-growing wood is east, descending metal is west and life-giving earth is at the centre.

ATTRIBUTES OF THE FIVE PHASES

Early Chinese thought gave each of the Five Phases some basic attributes.

BASIC ATTRIBUTES OF THE FIVE PHASES		
ELEMENT	FIRST ATTRIBUTE	SECOND ATTRIBUTE
Water	Soaks into the soil	Descends into the earth
Fire	Blazes with heat	Ascends into the air
Wood	Curved	Straight
Metal	Obeys	Is malleable
Earth	Receives (seeds)	Gives (crops)

However, this is only the beginning. As your understanding of the Five Phases deepens, you will start to see that more and more attributes are given to them and things become complex. Some of these further attributes are shown in the following table.

☯ **The Five Phases represent what ancient people saw in the world. They used them as a metaphor for the energy of life.**

	WATER	FIRE	WOOD	METAL	EARTH
Direction	North	South	East	West	Centre
Season	Winter	Summer	Spring	Autumn	Late summer / In-between seasons
Climate	Cold	Heat	Wind	Dryness	Dampness
Process	Storage	Flourishing / Growth	Birth	Harvesting	Trans-formation
Activity	Rest	Peaking	Initiation	Declining	Balance
Time	Night	Noon	Morning	Evening	Late afternoon
Colour	Blue / Black	Purple / Red	Green	White	Yellow / Gold
Sense organ	Ears	Tongue	Eyes	Nose	Mouth
Fluid	Urine	Sweat	Tears	Mucus	Saliva
Emotion	Fear	Joy	Anger	Grief	Worry
Numbers	2 and 6	3 and 7	4 and 8	1 and 9	5 and 10

FIVE PHASES AND FOUR SEASONS

The constant movement of energy as the wheel of the year slowly turns is one of the most compelling manifestations of yinyang and the Five Phases at work. However, you do not have to be a gifted mathematician to know that five does not go into four. This was a problem the ancient Chinese often came up against when trying to make the Five Phases fit with other systems that were based on the number four, not least the seasons of the year. The following subsections explain two ways in which they accommodated the discrepancy between phases and seasons.

A FIFTH SEASON

One approach was to insert a mini-season between the yin and yang halves of the year.

THE FIVE-SEASON YEAR		
SEASON	YINYANG	PHASE
Spring	Yang	Wood
Summer	Yang	Fire
Dividing season	Yin and yang	Earth
Autumn	Yin	Metal
Winter	Yin	Water

In some manuals using the Five Phases you will see earth connected to "late summer". This simply means that it divides yang from yin. It is a phase of transition.

TRANSITION PERIODS

The second way they dealt with the problem was to designate 18-day "transition periods" (土用) between each season. Like the dividing season in the first solution, these transition periods were connected to earth. In truth there was no new period. The last nine days of one season and the first nine days of the next were simply relabelled in order to accommodate earth in the cycle. The maths can be seen in the following table.

TRANSITION PERIODS		
SEASON	PHASE	NUMBER OF DAYS
Spring	Wood	72
Transition period	Earth	18
Summer	Fire	72
Transition period	Earth	18
Autumn	Metal	72
Transition period	Earth	18
Winter	Water	72
Transition period	Earth	18
Total: Four seasons	Total: Five Phases	Total: 360 days

Note that the traditional number of days in the Chinese year is 360 and not 365. This is why at points the Chinese had to adjust their calendar to make it fit with the astronomical year. They would insert larger months, smaller months or an extra month to make sure that the seasons kept in time with the earth's orbit of the sun, just as in the western calendar we have a leap year every four years to take account of the extra quarter day each year.

Remember these key calculations:

- 18 x 4 = 72 (the four sections of 18 earth or transition days)
- 72 x 5 = 360 (the four seasons of 72 days plus the 72 earth days)

Additional days are added to correct the calendar.

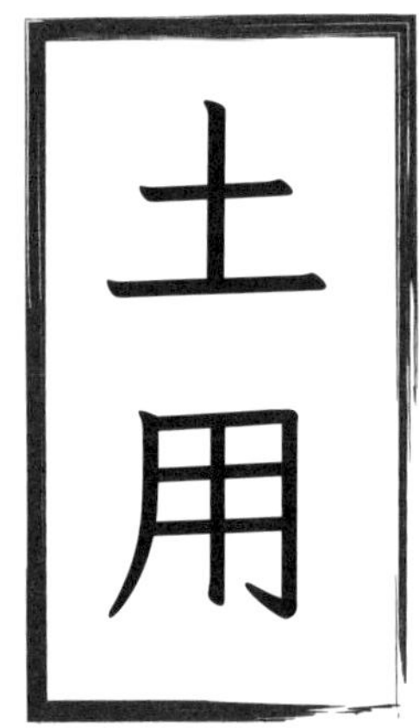

ABOVE: The ideograms used to represent the 18-day transition periods between seasons.

☯ **Whether in the form of an extra season or four transition periods, the earth element is the thread that connects the other four elements and seasons – from the icy chill of deep winter to the sweltering heat of high summer.**

TIMES OF DAY

Each phase has not only its own direction and its own season but also its own time of day.

THE FIVE PHASES: SEASON, DIRECTION AND TIME			
ELEMENT	SEASON	DIRECTION	TIME
Wood	Spring	East	3am–9am
Fire	Summer	South	9am–3pm
Metal	Autumn	West	3pm–9pm

THE FIVE PHASES: SEASON, DIRECTION AND TIME			
ELEMENT	SEASON	DIRECTION	TIME
Water	Winter	North	9pm–3am
Earth	Transition periods	Centre	Transition

Armed with the information in the table above, you can pinpoint, for example, that wood energy – that specific type of *chi* connected to the phases of wood – is at its most potent in spring, in the east, between 3am and 9am. And the chart below also tells you which zodiac animals are associated with different times of day, directions and elements. Note that in some systems the dragon, ram, dog and ox are connected to earth as "in-between" animals.

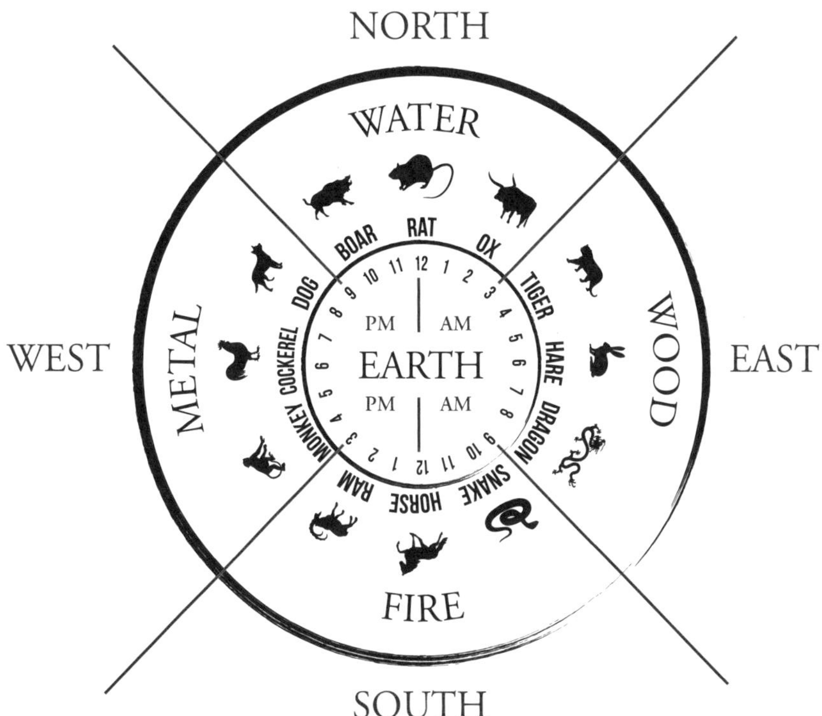

ABOVE: The times of day and their phases, animals and directions.

There are certain combinations of season, direction and timc of day when each of the five types of *chi* represented by the Five Phases are at their most potent.

THE FIVE PHASES AND YINYANG

The concepts of yinyang and the Five Phases were originally separate. Yinyang focused on rhythms in time and nature, whereas the Five Phases concentrated on natural elements. However, they have long been combined and are now considered to be inseparable.

The two systems progress alongside each other through the seasons of the year. The following cycle of life, from wood in the spring through to water in the winter, describes how the two systems interact with each other.

- Wood (yang) gives life to fire (yang).
- Fire enriches the earth (neutral).
- Earth (neutral) produces metal (yin).
- Metal (yin) produces water (yin).
- Water (yin) produces wood (yang).

As this process underlines, the Five Phases track the ebb and flow of yin and yang and it is yinyang-neutral earth that marks the transition point between yang at the end of summer and yin at the beginning of autumn. There are two ways to see this: one has earth in the centre of the seasons, the other has earth as a dividing point between the seasons.

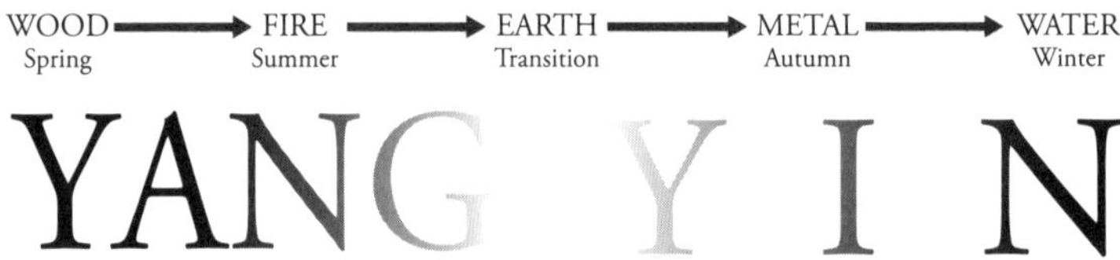

ABOVE: The Five Phases as they relate to yinyang.

Yang will always burn itself out and hand over to yin while it replenishes its energy.

A COSMOLOGICAL VIEW

We have seen the Five Phases depicted in various ways, including a circular diagram and a linear strip. Another helpful way to visualize them is in cosmological terms. The diagram below represents the elements as their symbolic representatives appear physically in nature. In the middle is earth, with wood and metal to each side because they exist on roughly the same horizontal plane (though wood is slightly above and metal slightly below). Below them is water, which trickles down into the earth, and above them is fire, which roars up toward the heavens.

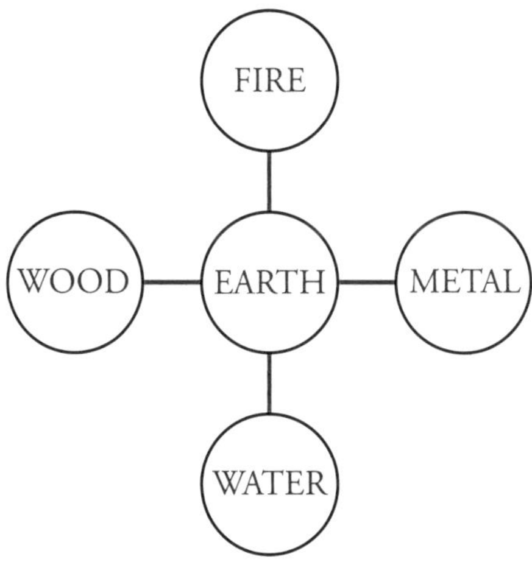

ABOVE: The Five Phases as they are positioned in nature.

Seeing the elements in their geographical positions helps us to appreciate that this system is a way to understand the physical reality of the world.

THE SIX CYCLES

Remember, the ideograms for the Five Phases mean "five" (五) and "movement" (行) – "the five that move". This is an important point, because we should always focus on the movement from one phase to the next, not on each individual phase. The relationship between the phases is everything.

There are six basic relationships between the phases. They are not complicated, but because of variations in translation they can often become confused. In the following list the six cycles have been named for their actions to help you retain them and to dispel any confusion.

THE CYCLE OF LIFE

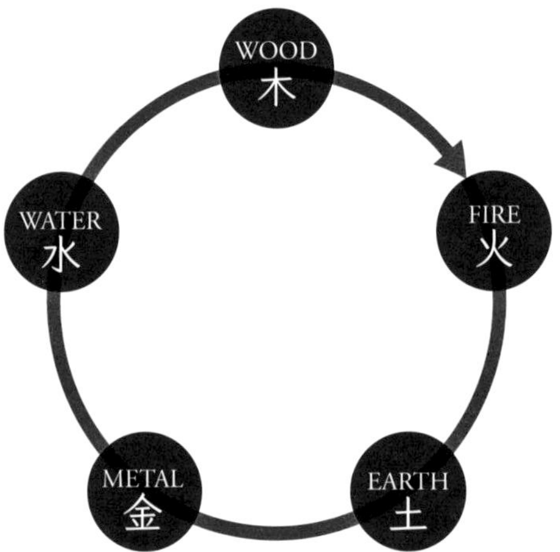

ABOVE: The cycle of life.

This is also called the "promotion cycle", the "generation cycle" or the "inter-promoting cycle". It shows that some aspects are born from or develop better when they are in connection to certain other aspects. For example, wood will make fire stronger and fire will enrich the earth. The basic outline is as follows:

- Wood generates fire, in the form of fuel.
- Fire generates earth, in the form of ashes that feed the soil.

- Earth generates metal, in the form of ore extracted from the ground.
- Metal generates water, in the form of dew forming on metal overnight (the Chinese saw this as metal producing water rather than as water vapour condensing on cold surfaces).
- Water generates wood, in the form of water sucked up by plant roots.

This can be viewed as a mother-and-child relationship because each phase "gives birth" to the next.

THE CYCLE OF WEAKENING

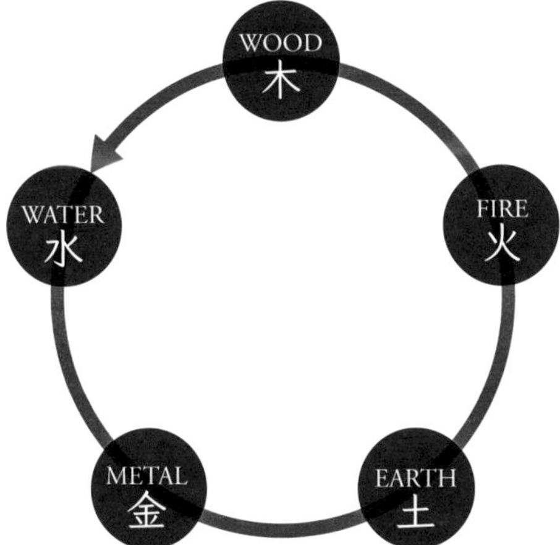

ABOVE: The cycle of weakening, which is the reverse of the cycle of life.

The cycle of weakening is directly linked to the cycle of life, in that when one element gives birth to another it is weakened because it gives up a part of itself. Essentially, it is the same relationship as the cycle of life, except that it looks at the interaction from the point of view of the "mother" rather than the "child". Unlike the cycle of life, which moves in a clockwise direction, the cycle of weakening moves anti-clockwise. The basic outline is:

- Wood depletes water.
- Water depletes metal.
- Metal depletes the earth.
- Earth depletes fire.
- Fire depletes wood.

THE CYCLE OF DEATH

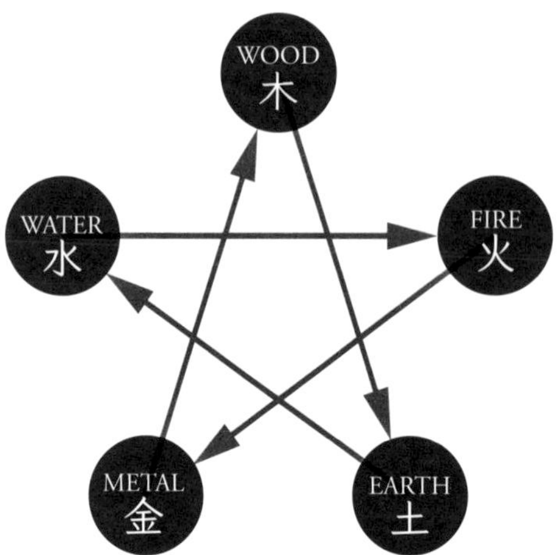

ABOVE: The cycle of death, in which each element "attacks" the next.

This is also called the "destruction cycle", the "conquering cycle" or the "controlling cycle". Rather than one element generating the next, here the elements work against each other. For example, wood in the form of a plough (in old China, ploughs were wooden) or a tree will churn up and disturb the earth. Similarly, the earth will soak water up. In this relationship there is an aggressor and a victim. The basic outline is:

- Wood conquers earth by ploughing it up.
- Earth conquers water by soaking it up.
- Water conquers fire by putting it out.
- Fire conquers metal by melting it.
- Metal conquers wood by chopping it down.

THE CYCLE OF STRENGTH

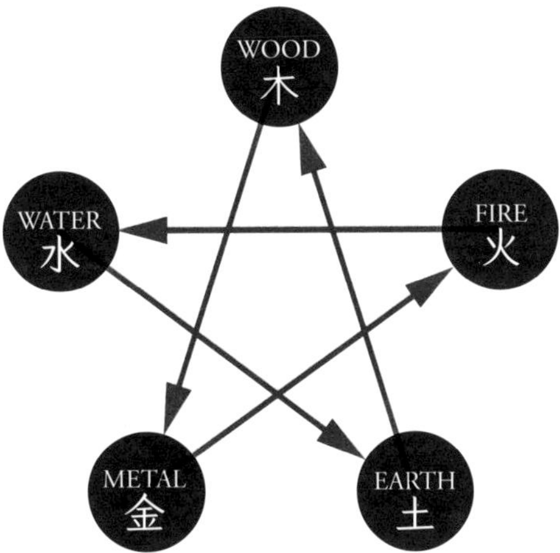

ABOVE: The cycle of strength, which can be seen as the failed cycle of death.

Just as the cycle of weakening is the reverse of the cycle of life, so the cycle of strength is the reverse of the cycle of death. Here one element has tried to attack another element, but it has not been able to conquer it because the element it has attacked is stronger. The basic outline is:

- Wood tries to destroy earth but the earth is too hard and breaks the wood.
- Earth tries to soak up water but there is so much water the ground floods.
- Water tries to douse fire but the fire is so strong that it evaporates the water.
- Fire tries to melt metal but it cannot get hot enough so it burns itself out.
- Metal tries to cut down wood but the tree is so large it blunts the axe.

THE CYCLE OF SUPPORT

The cycle of support is another reverse version of the cycle of death. However, this time, when one of the aspects attacks another, the aspect under attack seeks help from its friend to the left. Each element has a "best friend" who can "bully the bully", so to speak. This pattern is the same all the way around the circle. If you look at the cycle of life, you will notice that in each case the "victim" is the mother of the "friend", which is more powerful than the "attacker" and therefore the cycle of death is stopped by the cycle of support. For this cycle, each case has been illustrated with its own diagram for clarity.

Water fights back against earth

- Earth conquers water.
- Water generates wood.
- Wood controls earth.

Earth tries to attack water, but water uses its "friend", wood, to defeat earth.

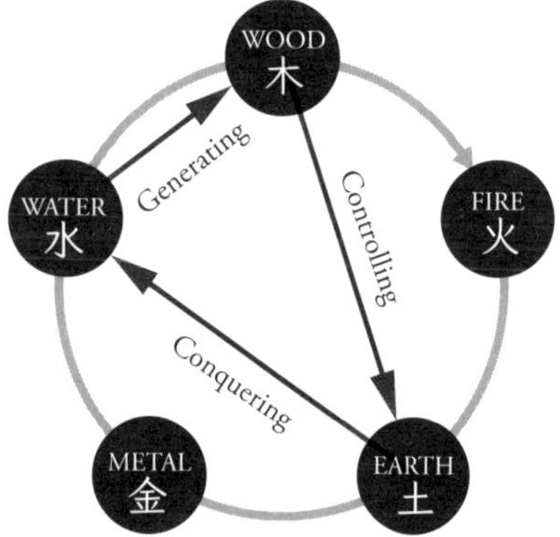

Metal fights back against fire

- Fire conquers metal.
- Metal generates water.
- Water controls fire.

Fire tries to attack metal, but metal uses its "friend", water, to defeat fire.

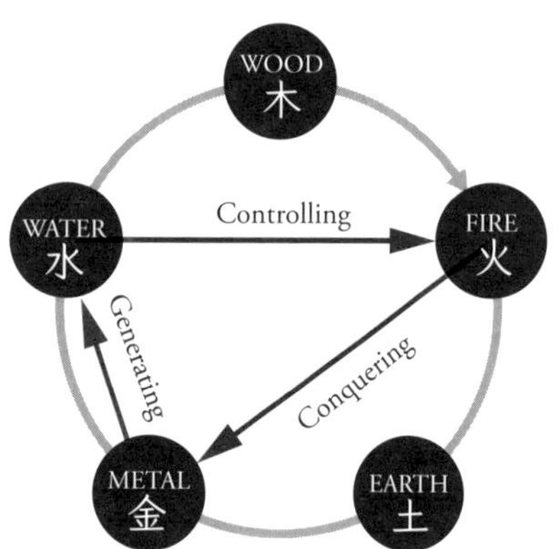

Wood fights back against metal

- Metal conquers wood.
- Wood generates fire.
- Fire controls metal.

Metal tries to attack wood, but wood uses its "friend", fire, to defeat metal.

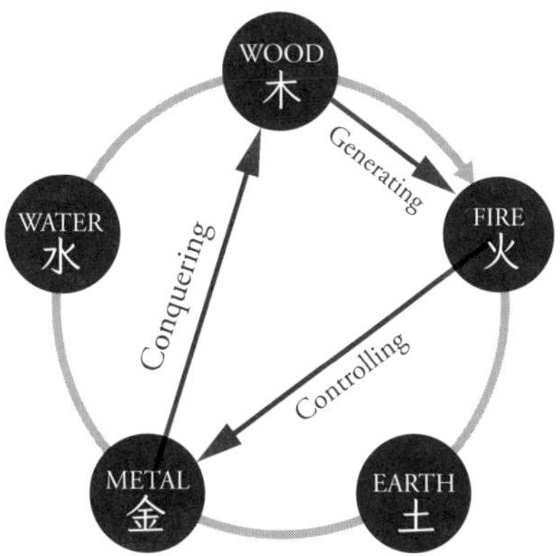

Fire fights back against water

- Water conquers fire.
- Fire generates earth.
- Earth controls water.

Water tries to attack fire, but fire uses its "friend", earth, to defeat water.

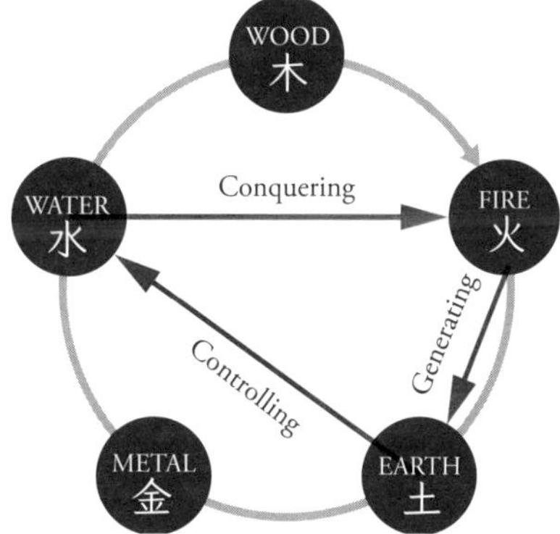

Earth fights back against wood

- Wood conquers earth.
- Earth generates metal.
- Metal controls wood.

Wood tries to attack earth, but earth uses its "friend", metal, to defeat wood.

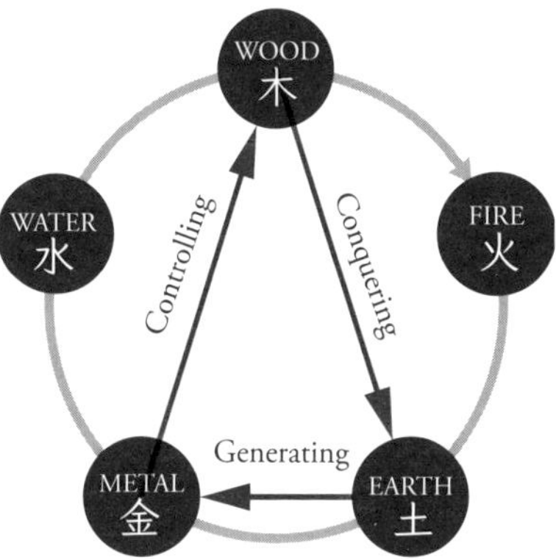

THE CYCLE OF TRANSFORMATION

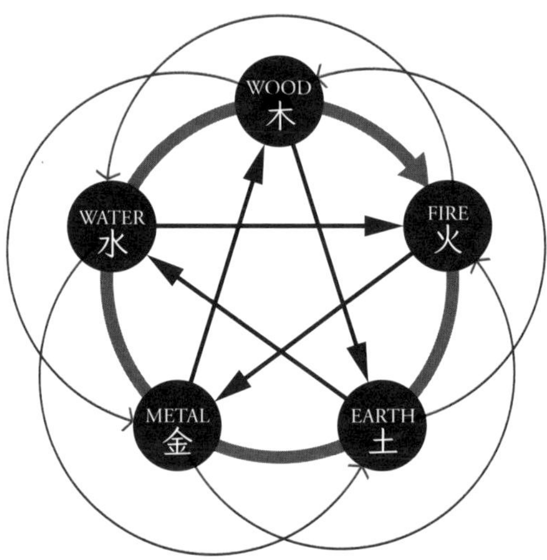

ABOVE: Instead of using the cycle of death, the attacking aspect uses the cycle of life to transform itself into its intended target.

In this cycle, the attacking element "knows" that it cannot defeat its intended "victim" in the cycle of death and therefore transforms into it instead. This is a two-step process of takeover based on the cycle of life. The basic outline is:

- Wood wants to destroy earth but it cannot, so it transforms into fire and then earth.
- Fire wants to destroy metal but it cannot, so it transforms into earth and then metal.
- Earth wants to destroy water but it cannot, so it transforms into metal and then water.
- Metal wants to destroy wood but it cannot, so it transforms into water and then wood.
- Water wants to destroy fire but it cannot, so it transforms into wood and then fire.

The cycles represent ways in which yin and yang *chi* can work together, be it in terms of the weather, the landscape, *feng shui*, Traditional Chinese Medicine and so on. The Five Phases are all about understanding the *chi* of something and using it to our advantage.

ALTERNATIVE VERSIONS OF THE FIVE PHASES

As we have seen, the whole system of the Five Phases developed over time and in different regions. This gave rise to variations, including the following examples. Although these are now seldom used, it is interesting to see evidence of how the theory evolved.

THE CYCLE OF DEATH THROUGH YINYANG

A different version of the cycle of death based on yinyang removes earth completely, because it is neutral in terms of yinyang. Above the earth the four elements move through the cycle of death alternating between yin and yang.

- Fire (yang) melts metal (yin).
- Metal (yin) chops down wood (yang).
- Wood (yang) soaks up water (yin).
- Water (yin) extinguishes fire (yang).

This alternative cycle of death highlights how the elements are just analogies to help people understand the way of nature – almost any order can be created but it is the underlying principle that is important.

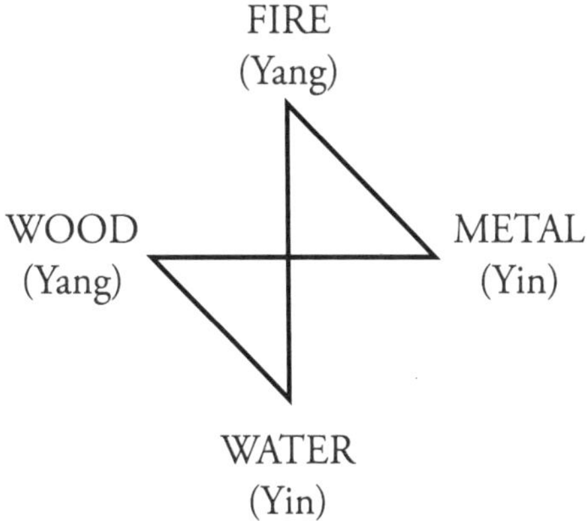

ABOVE: Starting at the top with fire, the cycle moves to metal, then wood, then water and then returns to fire.

THE FIVE PHASES WITH CLOUDS INSTEAD OF METAL

This different version of the Five Phases can be explained as follows:

- Earth allows wood to grow.
- Wood provides fuel for fire.
- Fire produces gas and clouds are gaseous.
- Clouds give rain which provides water.
- Water nourishes the earth.

A LINEAR VERSION OF THE FIVE PHASES

The following system is a linear process that starts with water and ends with earth. Therefore, it does not work as smoothly as the classic form, because it is not a cycle.

1. Water harmonises with earth.
2. Earth harmonises with fire.
3. Fire transforms metal.
4. Metal can control wood.
5. Wood decomposes and becomes earth.

☯ **The classic version of the Five Phases was not always in place. Before the theory formed into a single unified idea there were numerous variants, which are now seldom used.**

THE PRIMARY FUNCTIONS OF THE FIVE PHASES

The Five Phases are also given individual attributes that support their function within the world. Wood can be used to produce things, metal can be formed into tools of destruction, fire provides heat while water cools, and, below them all, the earth holds everything up.

FIVE PHASES AND ATTRIBUTES	
PHASE	ATTRIBUTE
Wood	Production
Metal	Destruction
Fire	Heating

FIVE PHASES AND ATTRIBUTES	
PHASE	ATTRIBUTE
Water	Cooling
Earth	Supporting

The earth supports the four major elements because the landscape is home to the other aspects of existence.

THE YIN OR YANG OF THE FIVE PHASES

Each of the Five Phases is connected to yin or yang or a mixture of the two. As can be seen in the table, wood is the highest aspect of yang. For this reason, it is sometimes positioned at the top in a circular diagram of the creation or destruction cycle.

FIVE PHASES AND YINYANG	
PHASE	YINYANG
Wood	High yang
Fire	Yang
Earth	Yin and yang
Metal	Yin
Water	High yin

The physical earth is associated with yin (and the sky with yang), but the earth element within the Five Phases has a balance of yin and yang because it is the foundation of all life. Note also that, although yang is at its strongest in summer, spring is given the status of high yang because this is the season when yang is bursting into growth.

Wood and fire are yang, metal and water are yin. Earth is a balance of the two.

NUMEROLOGY

For the purposes of numerology and multiple Chinese traditions, each of the Five Phases has two numbers associated with it: a basic first number from one to five and then as the cycle goes around again a second number from six to 10.

NUMERICAL VALUES OF THE FIVE PHASES			
CYCLE 1		CYCLE 2	
1	Water	6	Water
2	Fire	7	Fire
3	Wood	8	Wood
4	Metal	9	Metal
5	Earth	10	Earth

There is another system that allocates the numbers to yin and yang, but, as the following table shows, this does not match up with the Five Phases allocation.

NUMERICAL VALUES OF YIN AND YANG	
1	Yang
2	Yin
3	Yang
4	Yin

NUMERICAL VALUES OF YIN AND YANG	
5	Yang
6	Yin
7	Yang
8	Yin
9	Yang
10	N/A

The first thing to note is that in yinyang theory the number nine is seen as the highest number, so there is no allocation for 10. What is more, some of the numbers are seen as yang but are associated with a yin element, or vice versa. For example, the number one is yang but is also associated with water, which is a yin element.

☯ **Each of the Five Phases is associated with two numbers from one to 10 and the numbers one to nine are either yin or yang. These two numbering systems are completely separate.**

NATURAL DISASTERS

In traditional Chinese culture, disasters are seen as being the result of an imbalance of yin or yang within the Five Phases. When wood is forced against wood – for example, as trees rubbing against each other in a forest – the friction this causes can spark a fire. Wood is yang and an overabundance of yang can manifest as destructive yang – in this case, a forest fire. When fire is raging, it is in a yang phase. Any metal caught in the fire will become molten, making yin give way to yang. Yang is powerful and can defeat yin, but yin will return to dominance when yang has burned itself out.

☯ **In any subject an imbalance in the Five Phases will create problems.**

THE SIX FACTORS OF CREATION

There are either four or five actual elements or aspects, depending on whether earth is included. However, some people in ancient China thought that there were six aspects in total: water, fire, wood, metal and earth, as well as heaven. They saw water, fire, wood and metal as playing out their cycles of destruction and creation between mother earth and father sky.

Heaven
Wood — Fire — Metal — Water
Earth

ABOVE: The six factors of creation.

The concept of the six factors of creation includes heaven in addition to the four elements and earth included in the Five Phases.

PROPER HUMAN SOCIETY

As previously discussed, the second ideogram in *wuxing* (五行), the term we translate as the Five Phases, means movement and this movement can be either physical or psychological. The ideogram can also denote "human action", so *wuxing* can be translated as "the five ways to act". This looks at the right time to carry out certain actions and the importance of balance between different types of action. The actions are classified by element – so, for example, fishing and irrigation are associated with water, whereas cooking and the baking of clay for bricks are associated with fire.

The Five Phases in this context are the building blocks of civilized life on earth. If certain actions are taken to an extreme or carried out at the wrong time then civilization will fail, but if actions are balanced and allowed to flow in a cycle then civilization will flourish.

Humans can create a better society by carrying out actions associated with each of the Five Phases in balance and at the right times.

THE FIVE VIRTUES

There are five attitudes connected to the Five Phases. These are also often associated with the five virtues listed in Confucian thought. The following table shows those attitudes plus their connections to other aspects.

THE FIVE VIRTUES				
IDEOGRAM	CHINESE	JAPANESE	ENGLISH	PHASE
智	*Zhi*	*Chi*	Wisdom	Water
禮	*Li*	*Rei*	Courtesy	Fire
仁	*Ren*	*Jin*	Benevolence	Wood
義	*Yi*	*Gi*	Righteousness	Metal
信	*Xin*	*Shin*	Fidelity	Earth

☯ **If a person lives according to the five virtues of wisdom, courtesy, benevolence, righteousness and fidelity and understands the cycles of the Five Phases they will be a superior human.**

DEEPER MEANINGS FOUND WITHIN THE ORIGINAL CHINESE

The best translations of ancient Chinese texts give us a solid understanding of the theories contained within, but they invariably lose certain nuances that only Chinese speakers will understand.

Sometimes these nuances come in the form of wordplay through juxtaposing rhyming or similar-sounding words with different meanings. Although certain aspects of the language have evolved since these texts were written, a modern Chinese speaker will pick up on these examples of wordplay and smile in recognition. It is the same as a modern English speaker watching a play by Shakespeare and appreciating the dynamic layer added by the rhythms of Elizabethan verse.

Another example of linguistic subtlety particular to Chinese comes in the ideograms themselves. Ancient people built these up from the phenomena that they were observing, and when you can recognize this it fills your mind with an extra layer of beauty. A good example is the ideogram for "east" (東), which is a composite of the ideograms for "tree" (木) and "sun" (日) – meaning that east is the direction where the sun comes over the horizon with its rays shining through the trees.

A final example is the use of a word that has related but different connotations. We have already encountered this in the term *xing* (行), which forms part of *wuxing* (i.e. the Five Phases) and which has two main meanings:

1. ***Xing*** (行) – movement of the Five Phases
2. ***Xing*** (行) – characteristics of the mind (including the five Confucian virtues)

The subtlety is increased when one learns that there is another term *xing* represented by a different ideogram (星), which represents the five planets and their movements. The planets move in the same way that the Five Phases move, which in turn matches the movements of the mind. So this gives us three *xing*s, all of which are interconnected but independently mean different things depending on the ideogram and the context.

Even those who fully understand the whole system of yinyang theory may be able to find further layers of poetry hidden within the Chinese texts.

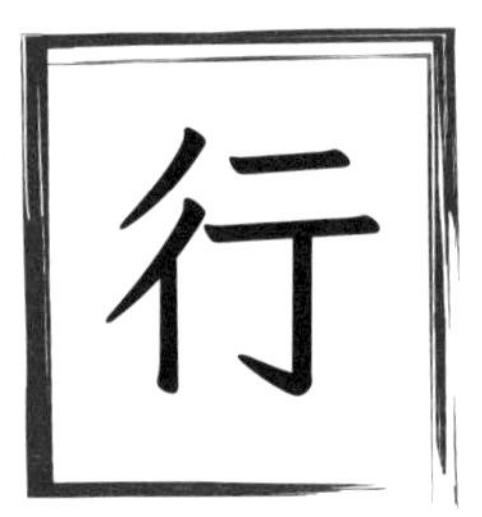

ABOVE: The ideogram for *xing* is fundamental to Chinese thinking. It encapsulates the movement of the mind, the universe and the Five Phases.

WORKING WITH YINYANG:
Understand the interaction of the Five Phases

By this point your view of yourself and your surroundings will have changed. You know now that you are more than just an individual alive in the world – you are a part of the great universal system that flows from the movement of yin and yang and is alive with the *chi* of the universe. You have now seen how the Five Phases – or the elements of water, fire, wood, metal and earth – are states of energy that interact with each other, providing the building blocks of the universe. These Five Phases manifest not just in the objects of the material world but also in the turning of the year and even within human behaviour and thought. There are interconnected relationships between everything and everyone. Look at your relationships and try to see how the Five Phases manifest within them, and if they are in a cycle of creation or one of destruction. For you to succeed in life, you need to identify and ride the rhythms of pulsating universal *chi* as it passes through the Five Phases of water, fire, wood, metal and earth.

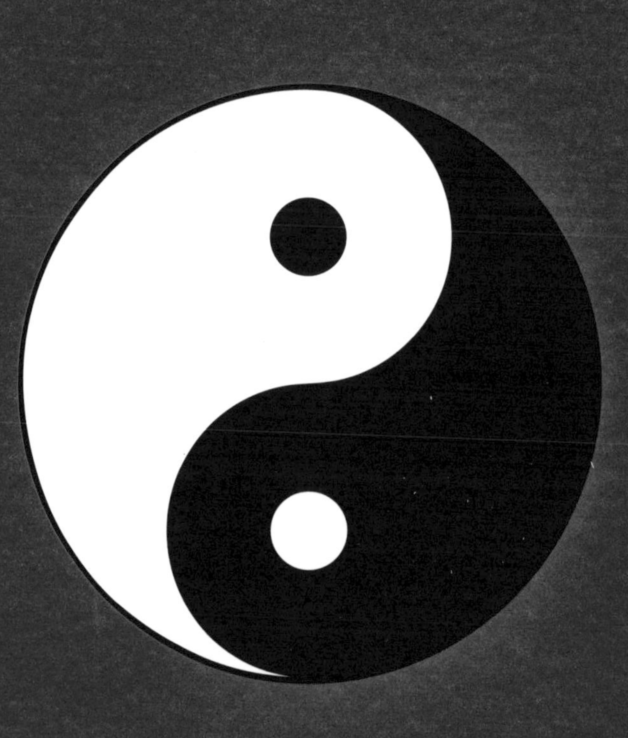

CHAPTER 17

TRADITIONAL CHINESE MEDICINE

TRADITIONAL CHINESE MEDICINE

The underlying principle of Traditional Chinese Medicine (TCM) is the proper regulation of the body through the correct flow of *chi* along channels called meridians and through good movement and diet. This chapter is not a course in Chinese medicine itself; it simply gives an overview of the fundamental role of yinyang in medical practice in ancient China. Today there are many avenues to follow to become adept in Chinese medicine. It is recommended that you do your best to find authentic tuition, but that you use the following to gain a grounding in a very complex subject.

MEDICINE IS A WAY OF LIFE, NOT A CURE

Doctors who practise TCM aim to *maintain* the body in a good state of health. Prevention through a well-balanced lifestyle is better than cure. In the modern western world, diets are often wholly incorrect and stress levels are high – factors that can lead to illness. In traditional eastern culture, the idea is to work with the energy of the seasons, eat wholesome and healthy food, be active and fit, enjoy a balance of work and relaxation and, especially in Daoism, lead a simple life.

When a person's health starts to move out of balance, traditional medicine recommends trying to regain a correct level of harmony before symptoms become too serious. Be aware, however, that treatments such as acupuncture or herbal remedies will not cure cancer, diabetes or heart disease. These are serious conditions for which you should seek orthodox medical treatment.

☯ **The principle of TCM is to live well and simply, keep on top of our well-being and regain harmony as soon as our health slips out of balance.**

STARTING WITH A GOOD FOUNDATION

In Chinese thought, correct balance of *chi* and yinyang is essential to well-being. This is expressed in the term *yinping-yangmi* (陰平陽秘), which means to have normal yin and a firm, deep base of yang. Most people are born with a perfect configuration of *chi*, but it is then our responsibility to maintain that balance. The Japanese samurai doctor Kaibara Ekiken said that everyone is born with a body built to last 100 years, but that each time we do something that is not in alignment with correct living we deduct some time from that life expectancy.

☯ Well-being starts with correct balance.

SCHOOLS OF MEDICINE

There are of course a vast number of different teachings and theories on healing from ancient China, and like most aspects of Chinese culture they became organized later on as traditions merged. Today TCM is more unified than it was, but there are still complex systems that sometimes differ in their interpretation of the principles. The following are just four examples of different schools and their theories.

THE SCHOOL OF COOLING

Founded by Liu Wansu (1110–1200), this school prescribed herbal remedies based on ingredients that cool excessive fire.

THE SCHOOL OF PURGATION

Founded by Zhang Congzheng (1156–1228), this school was founded on the idea that "evil" aspects create illness and that when evil impurities are removed from the body it will naturally restore itself to health.

THE SCHOOL OF THE SPLEEN AND STOMACH

Founded by Li Gao (1180–1251), this school held the idea that if you strengthen the spleen and the stomach then the body will regulate itself.

THE SCHOOL OF PROMOTING YIN

Founded by Zhu Danxi (1281–1358), this school was based on the idea that the body always has too much yang and that more yin is required when illness arises.

While different schools emphasize different approaches, the guiding principles of balance and moderation always hold true.

CAUSES OF ILLNESS

Illness according to yinyang theory is simply a problem of imbalance between yin and yang. However, before yinyang became prevalent there were believed to be four causes of illness:

- Heaven (possibly loss of the divine)
- Ghosts
- Bad behaviour
- Weather

The spiritual aspect of illness was very important. One of the original names for doctor in Chinese came from the name of a tool used by spirit-talkers in rituals to rid the patient of an illness by expelling the ghost that was causing the problem.

Yinyang theory took a much more modern approach to illness, seeing it as the result of one or more of the following factors:

- Emotional imbalance
- Physiological stress
- The environment

Even when theories of medicine based on yinyang became more popular, the old supernatural beliefs still persisted. Medicine in ancient China encompassed both a spiritual process involving exorcism and a complex analysis of the patient and their environment and mental health. This duality is seen in works such as *A Treatise on Pestilence* by the seventeenth-century physician Wu Youke, who put forward the idea that it was not the wind and rain that caused illness but a negative *chi* entering the body through the mouth.

In terms of the environment, there were believed to be six extreme conditions (*liuxie*) that can affect wellness if they are encountered for a prolonged period:

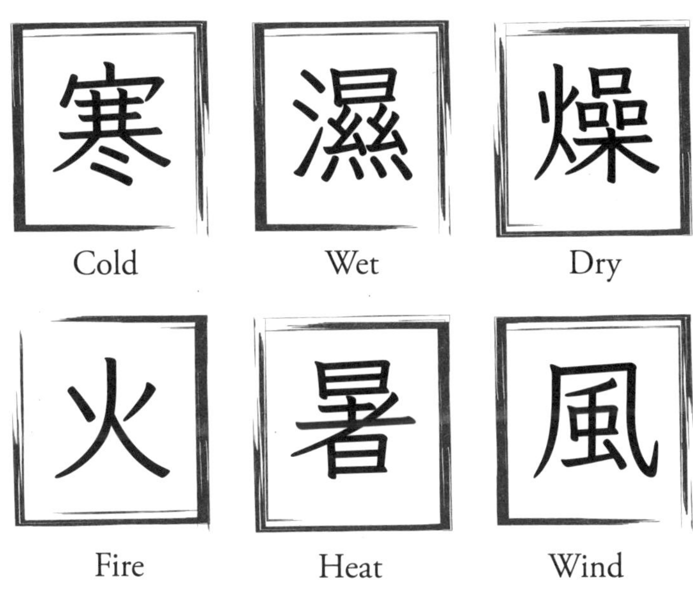

ABOVE: The six extreme conditions considered to be the start of all ill health in some forms of TCM.

Some aspects of TCM are in line with modern thinking, such as a connection between mental and physical health, while others show their origin in a tribal past, where the "doctor" defeats an illness through battle with evil spirits.

EXTERNAL OBSERVATION

In a TCM consultation, the practitioner will perform a basic observation of the patient, to include:

- Overall physical state
- Facial expressions
- Colour of the face
- Complexion of the face
- Shape of the tongue

- Colour of the tongue
- Surface of the tongue
- Sound of the voice
- Sound of breathing
- Sound of the digestive system

This visual examination may reveal a yin or yang problem. The following is an overview of ways in which yin and yang issues can be identified just from looking at a patient:

- Yellow and red colours imply yang and heat.
- Variations of blue imply yin and cold.
- Smooth and deep-coloured skin implies yang.
- Ashen and pale skin implies yin.
- Heavy and stressed breathing implies yang.
- Light and quiet breathing implies yin.

☯ **The starting point for a TCM practitioner is to observe the shape, condition, complexion, colour and sound of the patient's body.**

TI AND *YONG* – STRUCTURE AND FUNCTIONALITY

Each organ has a physical structure, which is known as its *ti* (體), and also a function, or *yong* (用). For example, the function of the heart is to pump blood, the muscles enable us to move, and so on. In TCM, a practitioner must account for and understand the structure and the function of each part of the body.

☯ **Each part of the body has both a form and a function.**

THE HUMAN BODY AND YINYANG

Just like all other things in the universe, the human body is divided into parts of yin and parts of yang. The body as a whole is divided into the exterior (yang) and the interior (yin) and the back (yang) and the front (yin). However, individual internal organs are either yin or yang and they may be divided into yin and yang subsections according to their position and function in relation to the other subsections.

As the table below shows, there are internal organs that store, which are called *zang* organs, and those that excrete, which are the *fu* organs. *Zang* and *fu* organs have their yin or yang designation, however that may change depending on the context. If there is not enough energy for the whole body, the *zang* organs will fight for resources and illness will start to develop.

THE HUMAN BODY		
BODY AREA	YINYANG	FIVE PHASES
Exterior	Yang	N/A
Interior	Yin	N/A
Back	Yang	N/A
Front	Yin	N/A
ZANG ORGANS (ORGANS THAT STORE)		
BODY AREA	YINYANG	FIVE PHASES
Heart / Heart protector	Yin	Fire
Lungs	Yin	Metal
Spleen	Yin	Earth
Kidney	Yin	Water
Liver	Yin	Wood

THE HUMAN BODY		
FU ORGANS (ORGANS THAT EXCRETE)		
BODY AREA	YINYANG	FIVE PHASES
Gallbladder	Yang	Wood
Stomach	Yang	Earth
Large intestine	Yang	Metal
Bladder	Yang	Water
Small intestine / Triple burner	Yang	Fire

The human body is divided into yin and yang areas and organs. In keeping with general yinyang theory, these classifications can change according to context.

THE TRIPLE BURNER

The triple burner (三焦) or triple heater is often considered as the sixth fu *organ. It is the area around the chest cavity and abdomen that holds the following three pairs of organs: the heart and lungs (upper), spleen and stomach (middle), and kidneys and bladder (lower). Unlike the other organs, it has no direct equivalent in western medicine, which can make it hard to understand and locate.*

THE THREE YINS AND THE THREE YANGS

Within the body there are three types of yin, known collectively as *sanyin* (三陰), "three yins", and three types of yang, known as *sanyang* (三陽), "three yangs". These can be divided into:

- Greater yin (*tai yin*)
- Lesser yin (*shao yin*)
- Declining or terminal yin (*jue yin*)
- Greater yang (*tai yang*)
- Lesser yang (*shao yang*)
- Bright yang (*yang ming*)

Each of the six aspects of yin and yang is associated with certain types of energy, months of the year and parts of the body.

GREATER YIN

- The start of yin growth
- The seventh month
- The eighth month
- The lung
- The spleen

LESSER YIN

- Yin in full movement
- The ninth month
- The tenth month
- The kidney
- The heart

DECLINING YIN

- Yin coming to a stop
- The eleventh month
- The twelfth month
- The area around the liver

LESSER YANG

- The start of yang growth
- The first month
- The second month
- The belly button (*dan*)
- The triple burner
- Gallbladder

GREATER YANG

- Flourishing yang
- The third month
- The fourth month
- The bladder
- The small intestines

BRIGHT YANG

- The strongest aspect of yang
- The fifth month
- The sixth month
- The stomach
- The large intestines

QUALITY, POSITION AND TIMING

As well as understanding the six subdivisions of *sanyin* and *sanyang*, a TCM practitioner also needs to be able to assess the nature of the *chi* according to the following three variables:

- ***Liang*** **(量)** – the quality of the yin or yang
- ***Wei*** **(位)** – the position of the yin or yang
- ***Shi*** **(時)** – the timing or rhythm of the yin or yang

☯ **The subdivisions of *sanyin* and *sanyang* create a complex web of interconnecting elements within the body where yinyang generates and collects. This is the foundation of understanding how to treat a person.**

> MONTHS OF THE YEAR
>
> *In old China the months were numbered up to 12. However, they do not correspond to western months. The first month starts at Chinese New Year, which normally falls in early February, so January roughly corresponds to the twelfth month, not the first. Do not try to match the western calendar to the old Chinese calendar; they are totally separate systems.*

THE HUMAN BODY AND THE UNIVERSE

Seeing humans as the highest beings in existence, the ancient Chinese used to correlate the human body to the world and the universe beyond in an attempt to understand their relationship to the unknown.

- The bones and flesh represent earth and soil.
- The eyes and ears represent the sun and moon.
- The top of the head represents the North Star (Polaris).
- Urine represents the waters of the world.
- The internal organs represent hills and valleys.
- Emotions represent *chi* energy.

☯ **The human body is a microcosm of the universe.**

THE FLUID AND THE STATIC

The body can also be divided into two basic aspects: the parts of heaven, which are fluid; and the parts of earth, which are static.

PARTS OF HEAVEN

- Blood
- *Chi*
- Other circulatory fluids such as lymph

PARTS OF EARTH

- Organs
- Bones
- Limbs
- Meridian lines

Fluid parts of the body are of heaven and fixed parts are of earth.

THE MERIDIANS

Meridians are invisible pathways that carry *chi* around the body in a single continuous loop. All along the meridian network there are hundreds of fixed points, like checkpoints or junctions, which are manipulated in therapies such as acupuncture and acupressure. This is done to ensure that there are no blockages along the meridian lines so that *chi* can flow smoothly.

To date, the existence of *chi* and the meridians has not been scientifically proven. However, they are an integral part of yinyang theory and TCM.

There are 14 basic meridians – 12 main lines and two more internal lines (the conception vessel and governing vessel). The main lines are all named after parts of the body. However, the names do not indicate the location of the meridians; instead they show more of a connection. The full list of the 14 meridians is as follows:

- Lung (肺)
- Large intestine (大腸)
- Stomach (胃)
- Spleen (脾)
- Heart (心)
- Small intestine (小肠)
- Urinary system (膀胱)

- Kidney (腎)
- Heart protector (心包)
- Triple heater (三焦)
- Gall bladder (膽)
- Liver (肝)
- Conception vessel (任脈)
- Governing vessel (督脈)

The meridians transport *chi* around the body in a continuous closed network. TCM seeks to unblock the meridians, where blockages occur, to ensure a correct flow of *chi*.

THE MERIDIANS AND TIME

Chi flow through the various meridians is said to have high and low points throughout the day. The following table shows at what time flow is at its most and least powerful in each meridian. Note that each meridian has its peak and trough 12 hours apart (for example, the lung meridian peaks at 3–5am and troughs at 3–5pm).

THE MERIDIANS AND TIME			
HOUR	TIME	MERIDIAN HIGH POINT	MERIDIAN LOW POINT
Tiger	3am–5am	Lung	Bladder
Hare	5am–7am	Large intestine	Kidney
Dragon	7am–9am	Stomach	Heart protector

THE MERIDIANS AND TIME			
HOUR	TIME	MERIDIAN HIGH POINT	MERIDIAN LOW POINT
Snake	9am–11am	Spleen	Triple heater
Horse	11am–1pm	Heart	Gall bladder
Ram	1pm–3pm	Small intestine	Liver
Monkey	3pm–5pm	Bladder	Lung
Cockerel	5pm–7pm	Kidney	Large intestine
Dog	7pm–9pm	Heart protector	Stomach
Boar	9pm–11pm	Triple heater	Spleen
Rat	11pm–1am	Gall bladder	Heart
Ox	1am–3am	Liver	Small intestine

☯ **Throughout the day energy flow through each meridian peaks and troughs in a regular pattern.**

EMOTIONS, ORGANS AND THE FIVE PHASES

According to TCM, certain basic emotions are associated with certain organs and also with the Five Phases of earth, fire, metal, water and wood. Emotional imbalance can cause problems with organs, which will lead to illness.

ASSOCIATIONS BETWEEN EMOTIONS, ORGANS AND THE FIVE PHASES			
FIVE PHASES	EMOTION	ORGAN	DIRECTION
Wood	Anger	Liver / Gallbladder	East
Fire	Joy	Heart / Small intestine	South
Earth	Worry	Spleen / Stomach	Centre
Metal	Grief	Lungs / Large intestine	West
Water	Fear	Kidneys / Bladder	North

Bear in mind that these basic emotions may be translated differently in different sources. There are also counter emotions, where one emotion moves into another in a cycle of feelings. (And to make things even more confusing you may come across alternative versions.) However, someone who is suffering from anger issues may need to be treated for liver problems, or the liver can be affected by an environment that pushes a person to anger. Likewise, worry can cause issues with the stomach, and so on. In this case joy or happiness can also be a problem. Overindulgence in any one emotion can lead to internal issues and a person's environment can lead to physical complications through psychological stress.

Consider the table opposite as a start point to discover more about how the Five Phases and emotions work together, but remember that translations differ, as do the teachings of various schools.

☯ **Emotional imbalance can affect the organs of the physical body and cause illness.**

COMBATING EMOTIONAL UNBALANCE

The emotions can affect the physical body. Too much anger damages yin, while an overflow of joy damages yang. With a balanced emotional state comes a healthy and balanced body.

There are four ways in which emotional distress can happen:

- Overindulgence in a yin emotion means less yang energy.
- Overindulgence in a yang emotion means less yin energy.
- A build-up of a yin emotion reduces yang energy.
- A build-up of a yang emotion reduces yin energy.

Here "overindulgence" implies conscious wallowing in a certain emotion, whereas "build-up" is an involuntary process where a suppressed emotion grows over time.

☯ **If you maintain a healthy mind and diet and keep up basic exercise, then a healthy life you will have.**

HOT AND COLD TREATMENTS

TCM treatments seek to rebalance and restore correct flow of yinyang. Because yang is hot and yin is cold, often treatment involves applying either heat or cold to counteract the effect of the overabundant element. This can be done by changing the ambient temperature or prescribing warming or cooling herbs or food. Of course, this is a simple idea: if a patient is burning up, place cold towels on them and serve cold drinks; if they are freezing, give them a hot water bottle and hot drinks. However, the principle goes well beyond this basic level. There is a whole array of yin and yang medicines, foods and herbs, each fulfilling a subtly different function.

Normally, a cold patient needs to be treated with heat and a hot patient needs to treated with cold. However, sometimes the opposite is true. In some yang conditions the build-up of heat is internal and not identifiable as externalized heat. Indeed, the internal excess of yang may create a knock-on effect and put a second position out of balance. This may cause a yin condition, which manifests itself as cold. So hidden yang heat can lead to visible yin cold.

In such a case, a cold person may need to be treated with cold in order to expel the hidden yang heat. Once the excess yang heat is gone the yin can return and flow correctly in the body, ending the cold illness. It is the exact opposite of what you would expect. Likewise, hidden yin cold can lead to visible yang heat, which requires a heat treatment to address the yin source of the problem.

There are four basic things to consider to help identify whether a patient's fundamental problem is one of yin or yang.

EXCESS OF YANG

If there is too much yang the body may show signs of heat and need to be cooled. In this case there is enough yin energy in the body but it is being overwhelmed by yang.

EXCESS OF YIN

If there is too much yin in the body it may show signs of coldness and need to be heated. In this case there is enough yang energy in the body but it is being overwhelmed by yin.

DEFICIENCY IN YIN

An underlying problem with a yin aspect may lead to a deficiency in yin energy, which can cause a cold disease. To treat this, yin has to be brought back to balance. It may appear that the body is too cold and heat is needed to treat it, but the problem is a lack of yin and therefore you should work on bringing yin energy back up to the level of the yang energy in the body. Adding more yang heat here is not the solution.

DEFICIENCY IN YANG

If there is not enough yang to run the yang aspects of the body, a yang disease may erupt. To treat this, yang function and levels need to be brought back to balance. It may appear that the body is too hot and cold is needed to treat it, but if the problem has been caused by a deficiency in yang, applying cold is the wrong thing to do.

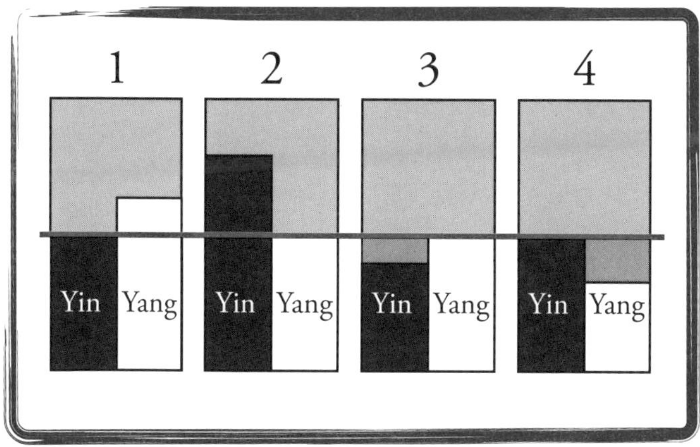

ABOVE: If yin or yang goes above the line of healthy balance (as in charts 1 and 2) you must expel the excess amount; but if there is a deficiency in either yin or yang (as in charts 3 and 4) you have to build up the lacking element not suppress it with its opposite.

The basic rule of thumb is that heat needs to be treated with cold and cold needs to be treated with heat – but in some cases the opposite is true. Visible yang heat can be the body's response to hidden yin cold, and vice versa.

THE BASIC TYPES OF TREATMENT

Most disorders in yinyang medicine can be attributed to one of the following three causes:

- There is the right amount of energy in the body overall, but either yin or yang is dominating the other.
- There is too much energy in the body.
- There is not enough energy in the body.

Each of these causes requires a different treatment approach:

- Yang should be treated with yin (or vice versa).
- Deficiency should be treated with an increase of what is lost.
- Excess should be treated by reducing the element that is too strong.

☯ **In yinyang medicine, treat with the opposite aspect, decrease an overabundant aspect or increase a deficient aspect.**

HERBALISM

The study of herb lore has been a major part of medicine in all parts of the world since the dawn of human history. Within TCM, herbs are typically used to get rid of parasites, to staunch the flow of blood from wounds, to supplement vitamins, to induce purgative vomiting, to regulate the body's *chi* and to cool down or warm up a patient.

It can take many years to master the subject, but below are the fundamental principles.

FOUR BASIC CLASSIFICATIONS FOR HERBS

- Hot
- Warm
- Cool
- Cold

HERB TASTES CONNECTED TO YIN

- Sour
- Bitter
- Salty

HERB TASTES CONNECTED TO YANG

- Pungent
- Sweet
- Bland

ASCENDING AND DESCENDING HERBS

- Herbs that have descending qualities are yin.
- Herbs that have ascending qualities are yang.

In TCM there are aspects of *chi* that ascend and aspects that descend. Certain herbs help in both cases, depending on the treatment the patient needs.

CONDENSING AND DISPERSING HERBS

- Herbs that have condensing qualities are yin.
- Herbs that have dispersing qualities are yang.

As with descending and ascending herbs, condensing and dispersing herbs help the body regain its correct balance of *chi* energy.

☯ **Herbs are yin or yang and they are used to bring the yinyang of the body back into balance.**

THE HUMAN PULSE

In TCM the pulse is all-important. Its rhythm is studied deeply and it can signal many things to the trained healer.

MALE AND FEMALE PULSES

According to Asian tradition, there are differences between male and female pulse signals. In older days it was considered bad for a man to have a female pulse and for a woman to have a male pulse. Yamamoto Tsunetomo, the author of the famous samurai scroll Hagakure, said that the peace-loving samurai of his day were becoming too feminine and that their pulses were changing from male to female.

SEASONAL PULSES

There are different pulses for each season. Each seasonal pulse feels different.

- **Spring** – akin to a string from a musical instrument
- **Summer** – akin to a hooking feeling
- **Autumn** – akin to the feel of stone
- **Winter** – akin to the feel of fur

PULSE OF DANGER

In samurai tradition a pulse can predict danger. Reaching up with your right hand, use two fingers to feel the pulse on the left of your neck and reach up with your left hand to feel the pulse of your right wrist – creating a form of triangle with your arms. If both pulses beat together all is well, but if they beat out of time with each other danger is close by.

 **Analyzing the pulse is an integral part of TCM.**

SHIATSU

Shiatsu is a Japanese form of massage based on the principles of yinyang. The term dates from the twentieth century, but its teachings are based on the older Japanese system of *anma*, which in turn comes from the Chinese *tui na*, which is based on Daoist ideas. As with other yinyang therapies, the premise of *shiatsu* is to regulate the flow of *chi* throughout the body and maintain a healthy balance of yin and yang. It does this by manipulating areas known as *tsubo*, which are collection points for *chi* along the meridians. A skilled *shiatsu* practitioner is able to balance out the parts which are lacking and the parts that are overabundant, creating equilibrium and health. The following sections give an overview of the system.

PREPARATION

A *shiatsu* practitioner prepares the room for treatment, they wear loose natural fibres and cover most of their skin to avoid accidental skin-to-skin contact with the patient, which can distract both people. Before the session they perform a series of stretches known as *makko-ho* and engage in meditation and energy exercises so that they are fully prepared.

WORKING FROM THE FLOOR

Shiatsu is done with the patient lying on the floor while the practitioner moves around them using their body to apply the techniques. It is not done on a raised table or on a chair. The point of working from the floor is to help both the patient and the practitioner to stay flexible, healthy and balanced. To do *shiatsu* in any other way reduces its effectiveness.

SHIATSU IN ACTION

Shiatsu in action involves the receiver adopting positions such as lying face down, lying face up, kneeling and sitting while the practitioner performs massage, joint stretching and body manipulation. Sometimes this involves vigorous thuds and deep pushing; at other times, gentle movements. The result is a looser body, more supple joints and a more balanced energy system.

DYNAMICS NOT STRENGTH

A common mistake in *shiatsu* is to apply the techniques too forcefully, but this soon results in exhaustion and can cause long-term finger joint problems for the practitioner. Practitioners should use natural movement and their body weight to apply the treatment – the hands are simply the point of contact between the two bodies, not the source of the pressure. The practitioner moves from the hips and focuses on the stomach (*hara*). From this point they pivot their mass around their centre to achieve the pressure they want through the hands and arms.

THE FOUR BASIC STYLES OF *SHIATSU*

There are four basic types of *shiatsu*, which originate in old China:

- **Basic massage (*pu tong an mo*)** – basic massage of the muscles but without any reference to yinyang and *chi*

- **Push and grab (*tui na an mo*)** – focused on fixing injury and with an understanding of yinyang, TCM and body structure

- **Pressing (*dian xue an mo*)** – detects *tsubo* depressions in the body and balances *chi*, the staple aspect of modern *shiatsu*

- ***Chi* method (*qi an mo*)** – an energy-based system like *reiki* and *qigong* healing focused on *chi* manipulation and projection through both touch and non-touch techniques

APPLICATION

Techniques are normally applied with the hands, particularly the palm. *Shiatsu* skills include:

- Support hand (while one hand works, the other hand remains on the body as a support)
- Palm overlap (placing one hand on top of the other)
- Circular motion (one hand on top of the other moving in circles)
- Shaking (as above, but shaking instead of rotating)
- Grasping (crossing over your arms and working outward)
- Double palm (interlocking fingers to make a single working palm)
- No touch (using the *chi* of the hands to warm the patient's skin without touching it)
- Fingertips (massage with the fingertips only)
- Thumbs (massage with the thumbs only)
- Clawing (dragging your hands in a tiger's claw over the patient's body)
- Dragon's mouth (massaging curved areas with the curved section of the hand between thumb and fingers)
- Fists (massage with clenched fists)
- Cupping (making a concave shape with your palms and then slapping the skin)
- Double-hand strikes (placing your own palms together to create an air pocket and then using the back of your hand to strike the body)

- Chopping (making small fast chops)
- Rolling (rolling the knuckles of the fist on the patient)
- Kneading (like you would knead bread)
- Use of forearms (massage with forearms)
- Use of elbows (massage with elbows)
- Use of knees (massage with knees)
- Use of feet (using your own feet on the feet and legs of the patient)

INSUBSTANTIAL AND SUBSTANTIAL

The concept of *kyojitsu* (虚実), "absent and present" or "insubstantial and substantial", is an important part of Asian thinking and *shiatsu* in particular. It means that there can be too little or too much of something. Within the practice of *shiatsu*, the following *kyojitsu* principles are important:

- *Kyo* is empty, *jitsu* is full.
- *Kyo* is the insubstantial, *jitsu* is the substantial.
- A lack of *chi* in one area can make the body manifest abundance elsewhere to try to combat the problem.
- *Kyo* is the problem, *jitsu* is the symptom.
- Sluggish energy flow through the meridians can be caused by a lack of *chi* or an excess of *chi*.
- *Kyo* is below the surface in a depression, *jitsu* pushes out of the surface.
- *Kyo* is hidden, *jitsu* is observable.
- *Kyo* reacts slowly, *jitsu* reacts quickly.

Pain in one area of the body can be the result of an issue elsewhere. *Shiatsu* focuses on the source of the problem (*kyo*), not the location of the pain (*jitsu*). If you find the cause and address it at the root, the manifestation will disappear.

SHIATSU IN YOUR LIFE

Shiatsu is thriving today. Think of it more as a way of enhancing well-being than as a cure for illness. While *shiatsu* does deal with injury, there is ample benefit in bringing *shiatsu* into your life as a way to keep healthy and understand the human body.

If you would like to find out more about Japanese *shiatsu*, see the excellent works of Chris Jarmey.

☯ ***Shiatsu*** **massage is about maintaining a healthy and balanced body so that yin and yang flow with ease.**

THE ELIXIR OF LIFE

Alchemy was the forerunner of modern science. One of its central objectives was to discover the elixir of life. In old China this coveted concoction was known as *waidan*. For many generations Daoist masters studied alchemical processes and even administered potions of immortality to emperors who wished to live forever (but unfortunately probably died soon after, of mercury poisoning).

Eventually, the Chinese came to accept that it was not possible to achieve immortality and so they moved their attention to supporting natural health through the principles of yinyang. However, the legendary elixir of life continues to fascinate to this day as the mythical "holy grail" of the yinyang world.

☯ **Yinyang is not a path to immortality, but it can help lead us to good health.**

A TALE OF IMMORTALITY

According to one legend, an ancient Daoist master and his two students formulated what they considered to be the elixir of life. However, in order to achieve everlasting life the subject first had to die and then be reborn as an immortal. The master and one of his students drank the potion and died there and then, but the second student fled in panic. A short while later the master and his student rose from the dead as immortals, and will continue to walk the earth for evermore.

THE FOUR ELEMENTS OF ALCHEMY

The four basic elements of Chinese alchemy are:

Heaven Earth Fire Water

These four elements are the primordial building blocks of the world. The list is almost identical to the original Greek elements of air, fire, earth and water, which suggests that alchemical knowledge may have been shared between the two cultures (although the extent to which this took place is unknown).

WORKING WITH YINYANG:

Explore TCM

Understand that yinyang does not only operate on the cosmic level and in nature, but also in the internal workings of your mind and body. The aim of this chapter was to lay out a basic framework of understanding so that you can step into the world of TCM fully aware of its complexity but not daunted by it. The hope is that understanding more about TCM will facilitate your journey into whichever system of well-being you wish to pursue.

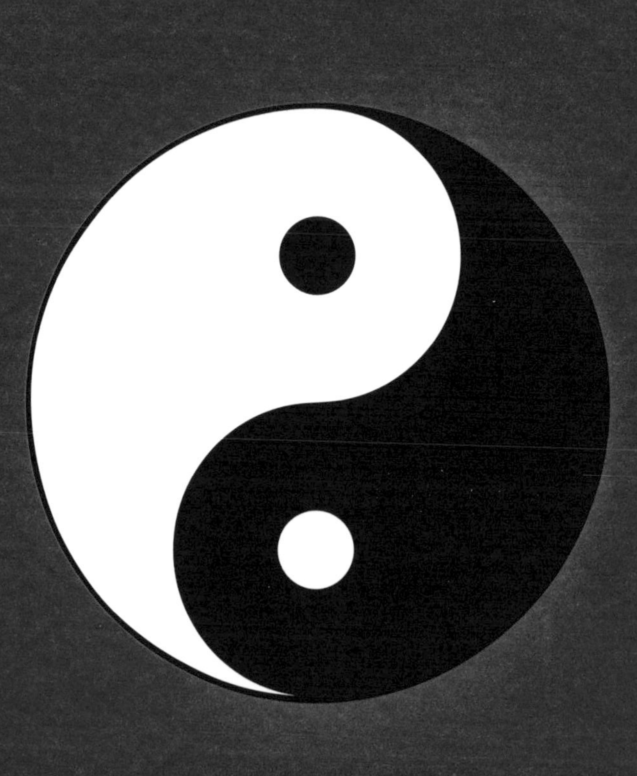

CHAPTER 18

THE HUMAN LEVEL

THE HUMAN LEVEL

In part 2 we looked at how society and yinyang interacted, and in this chapter we return to the human level. However, here we will look at how you can interact with yinyang, both as an individual and with a partner, to bring harmony to your life. This chapter has one foot in ancient Chinese society and the other foot in your own existence and experience on this planet. When following ancient ways you will always be partly in the past, partly in the now and partly looking to the future.

THE THREE PARTS OF A HUMAN

A human is made up of three distinct aspects:

- ***Xing*** – physical form
- ***Shen*** – divinity
- ***Chi*** – power or energy

The form is your body – it is given life through divine spark and it is powered by *chi* energy. In this way, we are like computers: a computer has physical components, its coding and software holds its intelligence, and it needs electricity to power it. When the *chi* expires, the body dies, the form returns to earth and the divinity divides into two aspects, one of which ascends and the other returns to the earth.

☯ **The human is made up of form, divine spark and energy, and when life is finished the three aspects separate.**

MUSIC

Music is said to be of the yang element (because it radiates out into the air), while ritual and dance are of the yin element. Therefore, to have music, ritual and dance in society brings harmony to all.

However, some historical texts say that music is a blend of yin and yang, which connects the yang *chi* of heaven to the yin *chi* of earth. Legend holds that the *guqin*, a five-stringed guitar-like instrument, was invented as a symbolic representation of yin and yang in harmony: both yang and yin types of wood are used to build it; the top section is considered yang (heaven), the bottom section is yin (earth); the length is 3 *chi*, 6 *cun* and 5 *fen* (just under 4 feet), which represents the 365 days of the year; and each part of the instrument can be divided into male and female, thus yin and yang. Chinese music as a whole can also be divided in two: the classic Chinese five-note scale and the more comprehensive 12-note scale.

☯ **Music and dance combine yin and yang energy, and ritual dance in groups promotes harmony.**

CONFLICTING CALENDARS

It is interesting to see in the symbolism of the guqin *that the Chinese did indeed understand that the earth took 365 days to orbit the sun. However, their old calendar system based on a 360-day year was still very much embedded in their traditional ways.*

DANCE

Legend says that musical instruments were invented in ancient days to calm the *chi* of unruly winds in the sky (yang). However, after this, the *chi* of the earth (yin) became too strong and all the waterways of the land were blocked up and water in the bodies of humans became stagnant so that people could not move well. To counter this problem, dance was invented so that people could regulate their bodies through movement. This is possibly the origin story of movement therapies such as *tai chi* and *qi gong*.

☯ **Different origin stories and theories have created a contradiction; some say dance and ritual movement is yang, while others say it is yin.**

MUSIC AS A SYMBOL OF GOVERNMENT

A common theme in the various systems of thought that competed for dominance in ancient China was how the people should be governed. One theory saw music as a representation of proper government.

- Proper government is akin to musicians playing in accord with each other.
- When all notes are in accord there is harmony in the "music" of society.
- When there is harmony the people are at peace.

Music is said to bring harmony. Music played a very important role within Chinese religion and often accompanies ritual, giving music divine significance as a symbol of the harmony of heaven and earth. When music is played and the people are in harmony, yin and yang also join in with this universal pattern of peace.

☯ **If a government can work together for the people just as an orchestra works together, then the people will be content and live in happiness.**

MUSIC AS A TRANSFER OF EMOTION

The Chinese also see music as a means for the player of the music to transfer their emotions to the listeners. This can be particularly powerful when a large number of people are listening. Ancient texts noted that soft music made people relax, vigorous music made people excited, and formal music made people righteous and respectful.

This principle of matching the music to the desired effect holds true today. Gentle music is played at train stations or wherever people have to be patient and wait in line; upbeat music before lively events like pop concerts; and dignified music like hymns or national anthems at formal events to make people stand up and be silent or sing patriotically.

☯ Music is the building of great works from a person's emotions. That emotion can travel to many others and change their hearts. This helps bring yin and yang into alignment so that humans can live in harmony.

ART

In art, yin is the subject to be painted, while yang is the painter. The subject sits in stillness (yin) while the painter is in motion (yang) and together they create balance between yin and yang. In the painting itself, strong bold areas are yang, while subtle and hidden or implied areas of the painting are yin. This is known as "yang strength" and "yin softness". It is not simply a matter of black and white; rather it is a case of strong parts and implied parts.

When assessing the yinyang qualities of a painting, you should consider factors such as the use of the brush, the shades of the ink, the weather depicted, the curvature of the landscape and whether the interior or exterior of a building is represented. The whole painting must be in harmony with a balance of substantial (實) and insubstantial (虛) elements.

The following list is a breakdown of yin and yang features within a painting:

- Light – yang
- Darkness – yin
- Exteriors – yang
- Interiors – yin
- Heights – yang
- Depths – yin
- Convex landscapes – yang
- Concave landscapes – yin

☯ Painting can be studied in terms of where yin and yang balance to create perfect harmony.

DREAMS

Even the dreams we have are a representation of our communication with yin and yang. Bad dreams can be a result of too much yin or too much yang energy. An old Chinese account gives the following outline for dreams:

- To dream of floods and water is to have too much yin.
- To dream of fire and heat is to have too much yang.
- To dream of killing or injuring people is to have too much yin and yang in the body.
- To dream in anger is to have a build-up of *chi* in the liver.
- To cry in a dream is to have a build-up of *chi* in the lungs.

Dreams like this can signal an imbalance of energy in the body that can lead to illness.

☯ Dreams reflect the state of your internal yin and yang. Recurring bad dreams can be a sign that your body is moving out of balance and heading toward illness.

CHI MOVEMENTS IN THE BODY

It is believed that *chi* moves to different places during the day and night and that yin and yang *chi* behave differently inside of your body:

- Yang *chi* moves to the outside of the body all day.
- Yin *chi* remains in the body.
- Yang *chi* rises in the morning.
- Yang *chi* is at full strength in the day.
- Yang *chi* lessens in the evening.
- Yang *chi* returns to the internal body at night so people can sleep.

Yin *chi* is therefore always internal and all types of *chi* return to the body during sleep.

☯ It is important to feel your natural peaks of energy and act in accordance with these rhythms. Yang *chi* in the body is stronger during the day and yin *chi* is stronger during the night.

DIVINATION

The ancient Chinese saw no paradox between the observation of the natural world and what we would consider the supernatural practice of divination, and yinyang was at the heart of both. Daoists believe that events on earth and in heaven are directly related to the social world of humans. A bad omen is said to predict the fall of a king, or a good omen the rise of a new leader. Likewise, earthquakes, storms and other natural disasters are considered as signs from heaven that human society is acting in an incorrect way.

Divination is an ancient skill, but it still holds fascination today. The principle was that a spirit-talker would formulate a yes/no question for the heavens to answer. The sun, the moon and other heavenly bodies were studied and any anomalies to their perceived natural order were read as omens. Other types of divination included burning tortoise shells or animal bones and "reading" the resulting cracks. One type of crack would signify "yes", another type would signify "no". These answers would be taken as advice from the gods and treated with great respect. The questions would typically relate to areas such as the suitability of a prospective marriage match or the likely outcome of a war, and so on. The following subsections are examples of divination in Chinese culture.

TORTOISE SHELL DIVINATION

The divination skill of *pu* is to make marks upon a tortoise shell and then burn it on a fire or apply heat and pressure to it directly using a hot brand or poker until the shell cracks. Following a previously agreed rationale, the type of crack is read as either "yes" or "no". The details of the rules do not matter, so long as heaven understands the system.

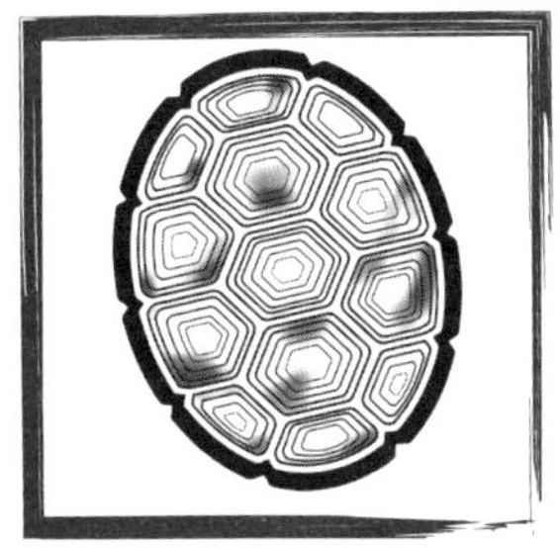

ABOVE: The tortoise shell, an important medium for divination.

STICK DIVINATION

Known as *wu*, this divination skill involves throwing or dividing sticks in various ways and reading their outcome. Sometimes the rattling of a container would bring out a specific stick, or elaborate ways of picking the stick or sticks would be used. The casting of the I-Ching can use either sticks or coins. The overall aim is to pick a stick that reveals an answer or to use the sticks to build a hexagram such as with the I-Ching (see chapter 9). To this day you can find such types of divination being practised in Asian temples, where for a small fee you can ask a question of the gods and receive an answer.

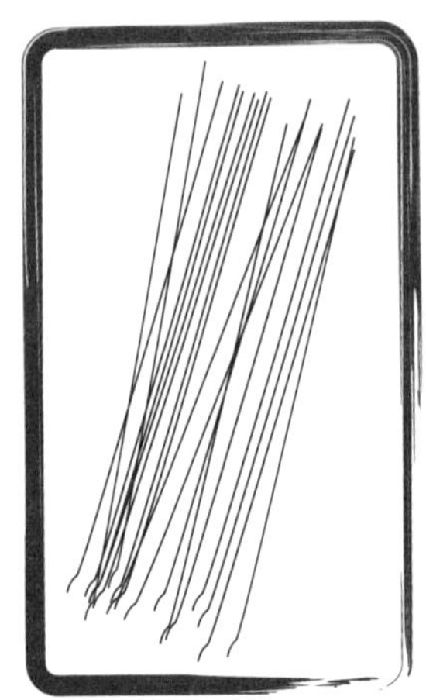

ABOVE: *Wu* – stick divination.

COIN DIVINATION

Coin divination is a simpler alternative to stick divination. It involves throwing coins in the air, allowing them to land, counting up how many coins landed on "heads" and how many landed on "tails" and then taking answers from the combinations. This quicker system is also often used to construct I-Ching hexagrams.

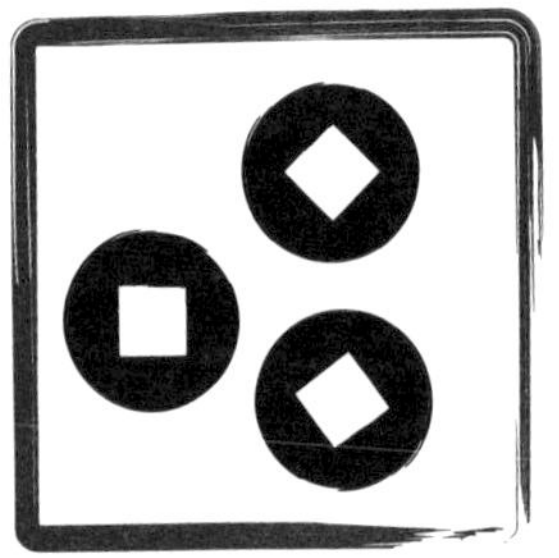

ABOVE: Chinese coins do not have heads and tails as our coins do, but they still have two readily distinguishable sides.

STAR DIVINATION

The studying, recording and interpretation of heavenly bodies was known as *douji* (鬥擊). One form of this divination focused on the direction in which the stars were facing, in particular the constellation of Ursa Major or the Big Dipper. Certain directions were considered auspicious or inauspicious. For example, the Japanese samurai referred to Hagun, the last star in the "handle" of Ursa Major, as the "star of defeat", because they believed that any army that fought in the direction of this star would be certain to lose.

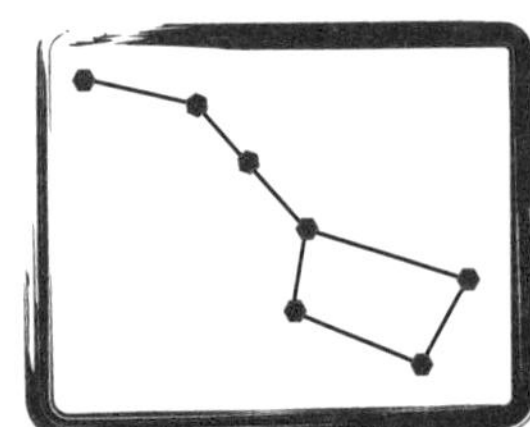

RIGHT: The Ursa Major constellation, with Hagun, the "star of defeat", at the end of the "handle".

☯ Divination is a part of ancient culture that still has sway even in the ultra-rational modern world.

PHYSIOGNOMY

Physiognomy (*mian xiang*) is the art of reading someone's character from their outward appearance. Often this is restricted to facial features, but sometimes it extends to the whole body. Sometimes the practice also includes an element of divination. It is thought that body reading originated in India and then spread westward to Europe and eastward to China and Japan. The ancient Greeks, for example, practised a similar system of divination.

Inspection should focus on angles, shapes, marks and so on, and when all aspects have been studied and identified, they are brought together to understand the nature (and possibly the future) of a person. The full array of a subject's tells and marks, both positive and negative, must be included in the analysis in order to gain an overall understanding of the person.

The following subsections give an overview of two of the main forms of physiognomy: face reading and palm reading.

MALE AND FEMALE

In some systems of full-body divination the heads of male subjects are the focus of analysis, whereas for female subjects the focus is the feet. This is because male is yang, which is associated with the upper reaches, and female is yin, which is associated with the lower reaches. However, generally there should be an analysis of the body as a whole for both men and women.

FACE READING

Certain face shapes have various meanings, and they are also connected to the Five Phases.

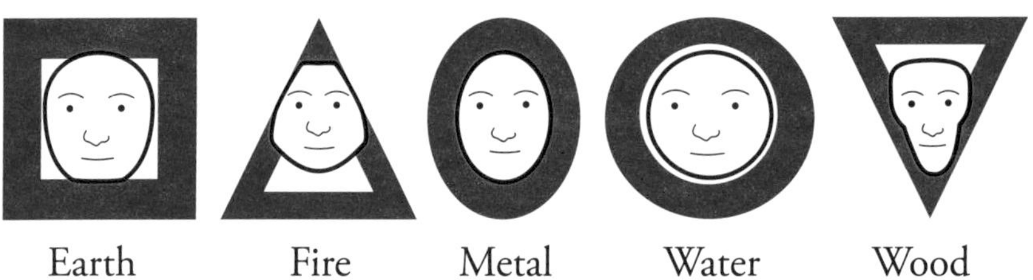

ABOVE: Face shapes and their associated element.

The face is broken up into bands so that it can be observed in accordance with the teachings of physiognomy. All the parts are also given names with Chinese ideograms. The system shown in the diagram below was taken from the Japanese ninja scroll Shoninki (1681), published as *True Path of the Ninja*, a central text of the samurai school known as Natori-Ryu. Therefore, these names are in Japanese not Chinese.

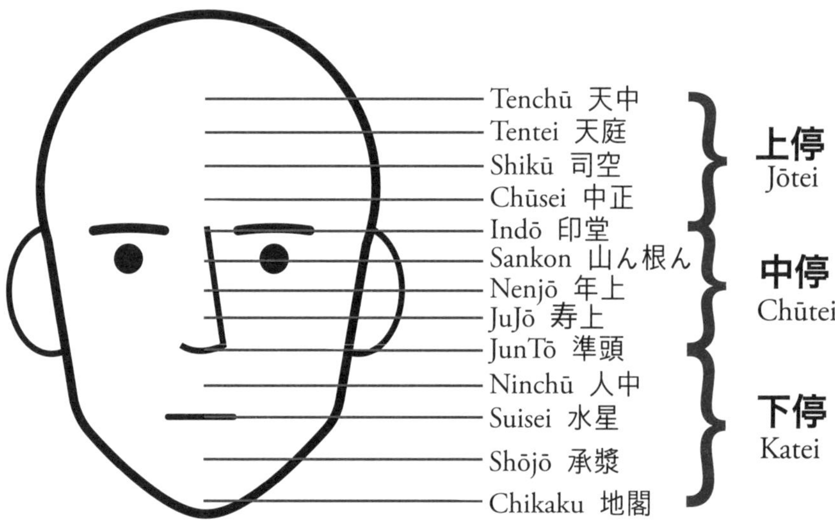

ABOVE: The parts of the face as itemized in the Japanese ninja scroll Shoninki.

BODY READING

The following list – again taken from the Shoninki scroll – is a simplified overview of the art of body reading. Note that it includes some advice on reading facial features as well as the rest of the body.

- A large head indicates a short but rich life.
- A small, elongated head means bad luck.
- A relatively short distance from the shoulders to the hips suggests a short life or an evil nature.
- Servants have bony bodies.
- Those whose head, torso and legs are all in proportion will have a good life.
- A full face with good flesh is a good sign.
- Wide nostrils mean shabbiness.
- Red lips and white teeth are a sign of good health.
- A straight nose is good.
- Clear eyes with bright white parts are a sign of good health.
- Good strong shoulders and a broad chest are good.
- A clear voice is positive.
- A large forehead is also good.
- Moles on the soles of the feet show a holy person.
- A deep navel is good.
- A thick moustache means long life.

- A fleshy and moist palm is a sign of good health.
- Many moles on the face is a bad sign.
- A mole between the eyebrows shows humility.
- A long tongue is a sign of good luck.
- There are bad and good lines on the palms of the hand.

This list is a reduced version and there are many other signs and body comparisons, as well as differences in interpretation between the various schools. The art of face and body reading is an interesting one, but requires a lot of study.

PALM READING

Palm reading, also known as palmistry, has a close connection to old China. Like other forms of physiognomy, it is believed to have started in India and moved both west to Greece and east to China, but the system was influenced by each culture, leading to a variety of traditions today.

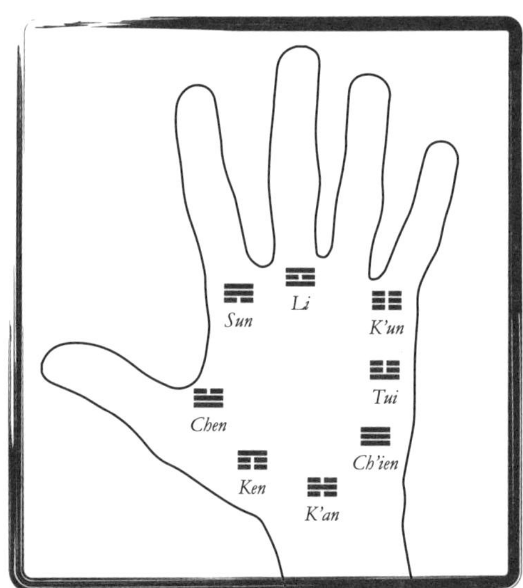

ABOVE: Palm reading can incorporate aspects of yinyang and the eight I-Ching trigrams.

Both palms should be read; one hand is known as the pre-natal hand, the other is the post-natal hand. This means that one hand has your destiny upon it, while the other contains the actions you will perform in life or explain how your life will be directed. In the West, the dominant hand (i.e. the hand you write with) is the one that describes your life and your future, while the other hand describes your potential. However, in the East a palm reader will always use the left hand as the dominant hand for men and the right hand for women, because left and male are both yang and right and female are both yin. It can also be conducted in conjunction with the principles of I-Ching.

☯ **The face, body and palms can be read to gain an insight into a person's character and destiny.**

FIVE ASPECTS OF RELATIONSHIPS

Relationships can be characterized according to five forms of interaction. These ideas appear throughout the book. However, they are collected here together with their ancient Chinese terms.

THE MOVABLE AND THE STOPPABLE

Maudun (矛盾) is the classic paradox of an unstoppable force meeting an immovable object. The teaching is exemplified in a Chinese story where a weapon-smith claims that he has made both an impenetrable shield and a spear that never fails to penetrate.

Of course, it is impossible for both these claims to be true and a relationship in which an unstoppable force comes up against an immovable object cannot exist either – not for long, at least. Sometimes you do need to hold firm, but at other times you need to give way – and the same is true for the other person.

☯ **Sometimes you may need to change your position within a relationship for it to work.**

ONE CANNOT EXIST WITHOUT THE OTHER

The term *xiangyi* (相依) represents the absolute interdependence of yin and yang. It is the understanding that one cannot exist without the other.

Hot and cold, tall and short, bright and dull, there must always be two sides. Even if one is more prominent than the other at a given time, this can never be to the exclusion of the other. Both must be there for context and comparison. Without both ends of a spectrum, there is no spectrum.

☯ **If you focus only on yourself in a relationship then the relationship will cease to exist.**

EACH EXISTS WITHIN THE OTHER

The concept of *huhan* (互含) is that each element always contains the other. This idea can be seen in the famous yinyang symbol. Yinyang works on potential; even the most powerful yang element holds a small amount of yin and the balance will eventually swing back toward yin. The seed of the future is always found in the present.

☯ **One person is never completely yang nor the other completely yin, and the balance of power moves from one person to the other and back again.**

ACTION AND REACTION

Jiaogan (交感) is the idea that if one part moves, the other must also move. When yin grows, yang decreases; when yang grows, yin decreases. Always remember, when you make a move of any kind it changes those you are in a relationship with, including heaven and the Dao.

☯ **Your actions affect the people closest to you.**

MUTUAL SUPPORT

Known as *hubu* (互補), this represents the idea that yin and yang support each other. Even when one is more powerful, it does not lord its power over the other. They are always in harmony within any situation and work together to create whatever is needed.

☯ **Two people working together harmoniously can achieve more than twice as much as one person.**

LEADERSHIP IN RELATIONSHIPS

Yinyang represents the way harmony can be found within a relationship; this is also echoed in Confucianism. The three traditional types of relationship described in yinyang theory are:

- **Leader (yang)** – follower (yin)
- **Parent (yang)** – child (yin)
- **Husband (yang)** – wife (yin)

Be careful here. These relationship patterns do not automatically mean that yang dominates yin and that yin is always subordinate. While yang is in a leadership position, yin helps develop the power of yang by participating in a harmonious relationship. Of course, a leader and a parent are figures of authority and *historically* husbands were dominant over their wives. In Asia, often the man governs the direction of the family while the woman manages the household. Remember, though, that in all situations there is the dominant and the submissive, even though those roles may change if the situation changes.

☯ **Yang energy leads, but when it is spent, yin energy takes over so that yang can regenerate itself.**

WHEN TO MARRY

A man and a woman should marry in spring, because this is when yang is on the rise and the high yin energy of winter intermingles and flows with the high yang energy of spring. Spring is the perfect time for the mixing of yin and yang in harmony. Weddings should take place in spring because this is when male and female energy mix the best.

YINYANG AND SEX

Sex is an important way in which humans can manipulate yin and yang and gain power from the Way. China has a form of "sex magic", a term which translates as something like "the art of the bedroom". In yinyang theory, the main purpose of sex is to promote proper cultivation of *chi*, leading to good physical and mental health and cosmic harmony. However, sex must be done in the proper manner if increased life force and longevity are to be the result. If one follows the principles of yinyang as laid out in serious studies on sex by Daoist masters, a man and a woman can act out the roles of heaven and earth when they have sex. The following subsections summarize the key principles.

☯ **In ancient China, to give sex was yang and to receive sex was yin.**

PROPER MENTAL ATTITUDE

The male (or yang) partner must be calm and unrushed, not over eager but still and reserved. He must attain the following three states:

- Settled *chi*
- Settled emotions (heart)
- Pure intention

These three together comprise the attitude required to create cosmic sex. The female (yin) partner should bathe in the yin energy being generated.

☯ **The yang partner must take second place in sex and hold themselves back.**

THE FEMALE ORGASM

The yang partner should withhold himself until the yin partner has reached multiple orgasms. Sperm is of the yang element and to spend it too soon will cause a man to lose energy. The more orgasms a woman has the more yin energy is generated, filling both partners with power.

☯ **A woman's orgasm replenishes the man with yin energy.**

SEX AS A BATTLE

A man should regard sex as a battle, in which the objective is to collect "loot" in the form of yin energy. The more yin-generating orgasms the woman has, the greater the man's victory; but if he ejaculates before the woman has any orgasms, the battle is lost.

For a woman, sex is a means to have pleasure and bring yin energy into the world. For the man, it is about taking that yin energy to supplement his yang. However, too much sex leads to a loss of vital internal energy and in some cases, the withholding of sex is also a way to build up energy reserves.

For a man to win the battle of sex he must give a woman as many orgasms as possible so that he can "steal" all of the extra yin energy she generates.

LANGUAGE OF LOVE

In old Chinese texts about sex, the word for penis translates literally as the "tool of yang", while the vagina is the "house of yin". The term for sex itself translates as "collecting yin energy".

THE EIGHT BENEFITS OF SEX

According to sex scholars of ancient China, sex brings eight benefits:

- Creates stronger sperm
- Collects *chi*
- Increases internal organ vitality
- Builds strong bones
- Promotes good circulation
- Improves blood quality
- Increases fluids
- Regulates the body

Sex is not only a means of reproduction but a way to benefit the whole body.

THE THREE REASONS TO HAVE GOOD SEX

In addition to the eight physical benefits mentioned previously, having good sex confers three universal benefits. If both partners have sex mindfully, with focus and concentration, they will both benefit. Also, from a spiritual aspect, sex is a union with the cosmos through yin and yang. Therefore, sex done correctly does the following:

- Creates a healthy body
- Unifies the spirit
- Engages with cosmic forces

Sex is a cosmic ritual played out on earth. Do not see sex as being just for pleasure or procreation; see it as a way to communicate with the Dao and promote a healthier life.

☯ **In unifying yin and yang, sex represents a cosmic ritual.**

THE TWO ASPECTS OF THE SOUL

Moving on from human life and love we come to human death, when a person's *chi* either diminishes or breaks up and returns to the Dao. It is not clear whether our *chi* leaves us at death, or whether it loses all its power, or whether the bonds that have held us in place as a human break down and the *chi* divides again. Such questions are a topic of debate for the modern yinyang scholar and the answers are not simple.

The soul or spirit in China is divided into two parts:

- ***Hun* (魂)** – the yang element connected to the sky or heaven
- ***Po* (魄)** – the yin element connected to the earth

Each person's identity and personality combine aspects of heaven and earth, but when the person dies the two aspects divide and return to their origin. *Hun*, the "cloud spirit", flies quickly up into the sky, while *po*, the "white spirit", lingers around the body and tomb for a long time before descending into the earth. *Hun* may turn into a god or become an unseen spirit (神) in "heaven", while *po* may become an earthbound ghost known as a *gui* (鬼). In old burial practices, the tomb was known as the "house of yin" and was the place where the *po* aspect of the soul could reside, whereas a house for the living was called a "house of yang".

The origin of the word *po* is very old. It possibly means the growing light of a new moon. However, later it came to mean the bright part of the soul that returns to earth after death. Remember that the moon and the earth are both aspects of yin, so the link between moon and earth represented by *po* carries a powerful connection to yin.

To make things more complex, there are three *hun* and seven *po* subcategories, each of which connects to yin and yang in different ways.

What is more, there are actually five aspects of the soul in Chinese lore (see page 13). However, here we will deal with the parts primarily connected to yin and yang.

THE CHINESE DAY OF THE DEAD

The traditional Chinese day of the dead is on the fifteenth day of the seventh month in the Chinese calendar. This day is specifically for celebrating the po *(yin) aspect of the soul, the part that has remained on earth and not ascended into heaven. Communities gather to light lanterns for the dead and engage in ritual dancing.*

Remember, this is in the Chinese calendar and is therefore not 15 July, but is a date that will always fall later – in the seventh month after Chinese New Year. However, be aware that some Asian countries have now adopted the western calendar and no longer celebrate on the correct day.

ASPECTS OF *HUN*

The following are aspects connected to the idea of *hun* or sky spirit:

- Breathing
- Brightness
- Consciousness
- Intelligence
- Vitality
- Volatility

ASPECTS OF *PO*

The following are aspects connected to the idea of *po* or earth spirit:

- Eating
- Heaviness
- Physical body
- Restraint
- Strength
- Virtue

Hun and *po* merge to form the human body and soul. If we have a proper understanding of yin and yang and correct actions as a human, these two divine forces will allow us to lead a full life and they will only separate at death.

BEHIND THE VEIL OF LIFE

The ideogram for spirit in Chinese (神) actually means "that which is unseen or behind the veil of reality". In Japanese, it is the ideogram used to represent kami, the gods of Shinto and dead ancestors. In yinyang theory these spirits, or shen, *are in heaven and inspire humans in their lives.*

The ideograms known as shenming *(神明) refer to "bright spirits". This can mean spirits beyond the veil of life or the bright spirit of your own nature.*

THE JOURNEY OF THE SOUL

As we have seen, *hun* is yang and wants to return to the sky, while *po* is yin and wants to go back into the ground. From there they continue on with the journey of existence with the goal of reaching back to the source of the universe. However, they can only do this if the person who has died has cultivated enough life force during their lifetime to fuel this two-pronged journey of the soul. If the person uses up every last "drop" of *chi*, upon death the two aspects of the soul disintegrate and do not form into anything.

This part of the story of the soul can be confusing if we think about it using western logic. How can there be any *chi* left over when a person has died? Surely our *chi* gauge is registering zero at this point? In which case, what is there to stop us being blinked out of existence? The only answer to these questions is to live correctly and trust in the Dao.

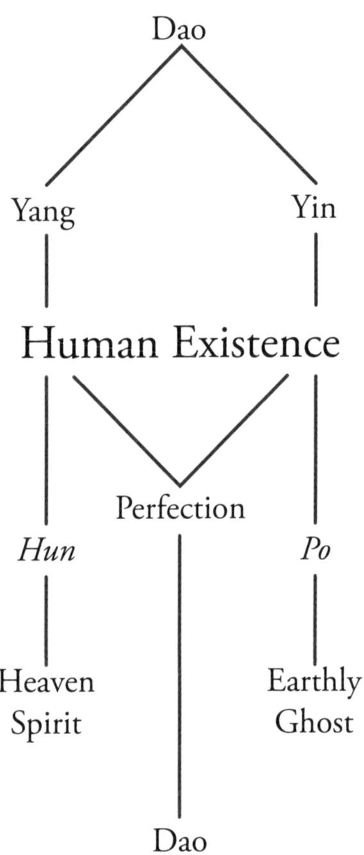

ABOVE: A diagram showing how human existence is related to yin and yang, *po* and *hun* and, ultimately, the Dao.

***Hun*, the yang part of the soul, ascends to heaven after death, while *po*, the yin part, remains with the body before descending into the earth.**

THE LIVING AND THE DEAD

Yinyang is also a relationship between the living and the dead. The living, who are yang, should be supported and enriched, while the dead, who are yin, should be honoured and venerated. Supporting each other in life is a yang aspect; just as wood supports fire by being its fuel, so people support each other. When the ancients threw sacred metal objects (yin) into water (yin), they were paying respects to the dead in a way that doubled up on the power of yin.

The living and the dead are in a relationship. The living honour the dead with offerings and prayer; the dead watch over the living.

WORKING WITH YINYANG:

Try the ancient ways

While most of the concepts and practices covered in this chapter are from ancient China, they can still be a part of your own life. Engage with art, interpret your dreams, observe how emotions can be transferred through music and how divination can help you tell the future, treat sex as a cosmic ritual, and maintain your connection to the dead. Know that your own spirit will move on to a higher level if you perfect the system laid out by yinyang theory and follow the Dao.

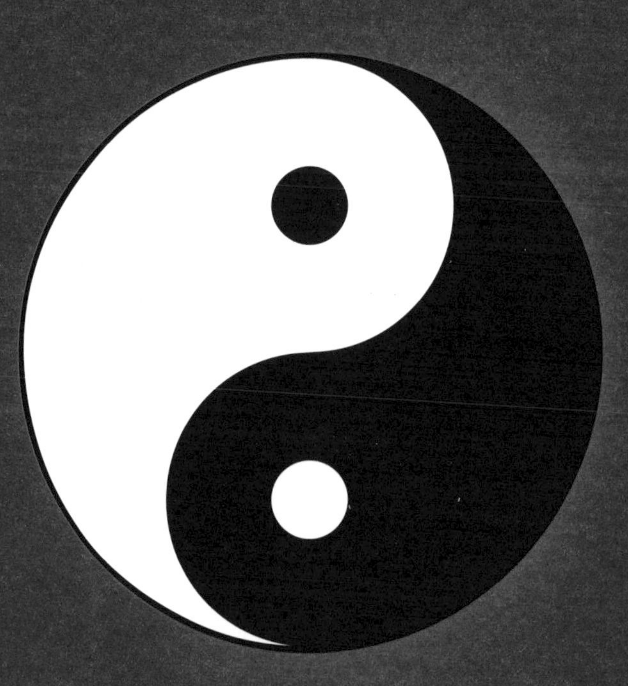

CHAPTER 19

LIVING THE YINYANG WAY

LIVING THE YINYANG WAY

Throughout this book we have been looking at how the world works according to yinyang theory; now in this chapter you will learn how to use yinyang to make the world work for you. While it is important to know how the universe came to be and how to recognize the patterns of nature which flow around you, it is also important to know how to ride those waves and to harvest from those patterns. It is not a negative act to take from the world – the world is there to be enjoyed. However, it is wrong to take too much, to push nature to the edge of ruin and society to the brink of chaos. Your goal is to be in the correct place, at the correct time, doing the correct thing and having the wisdom to know when you have enough to satisfy you.

STEALING FROM THE WAY

To start building a deeper relationship with the Way, consider the story of the rich man and the thief. According to this legend a poor man asked a rich man how he had managed to become so rich, to which the rich man replied that he had done so by stealing.

The poor man, misunderstanding the rich man's true meaning, started to steal from other people. After a while he was caught and punished, so he returned to the rich man to ask him what he had done wrong. The rich man told him that he should never steal from people but that instead he should steal from heaven.

The poor man was perplexed by this answer and so sought out a master to explain what the rich man had meant. The master explained that life is about empowering yourself with yin and yang and that all human bounty comes from a true alignment with the principles of heaven.

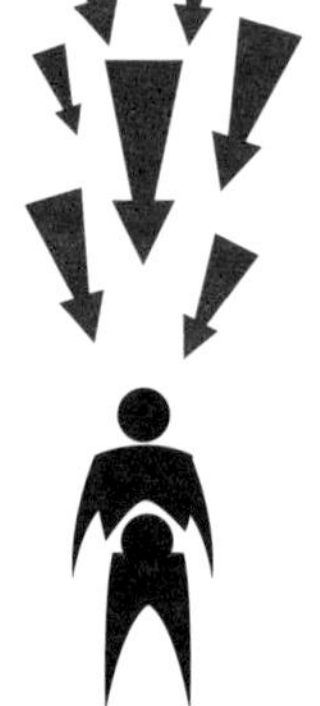

ABOVE: The Dao has more than enough for all life in the universe, so long as we take only what we need.

This story hinges on a play on words in Chinese. As we have already learned, the term *Dao* (道) means "the Way", but there is another word *dao* (盗) with the same pronunciation that means "to steal". This is where the idea of "stealing from the Way" comes from. The point the rich man is making is that by aligning himself correctly with the principles of heaven and leading a pure life he has placed himself in a situation that yields continuous bounty from heaven without taking from other humans. The Dao rewards him with what he needs.

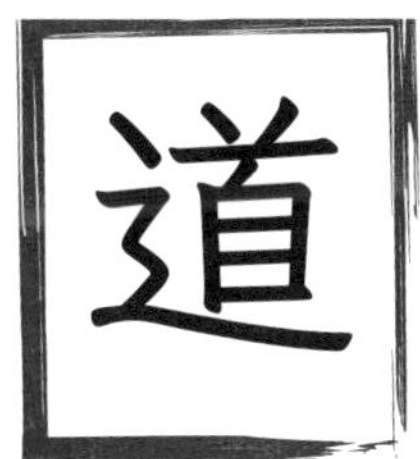

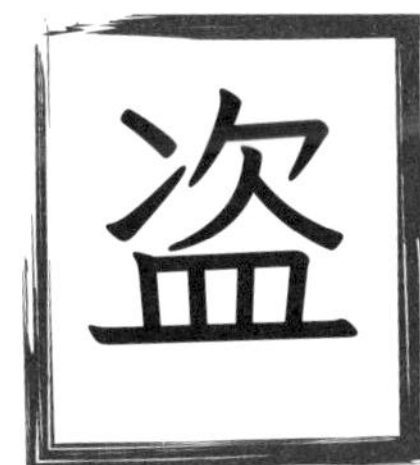

ABOVE: The ideograms representing the two meanings of *dao*: the eternal Way (left) and a verb meaning to steal or take (right).

Do not become bogged down in the negative connotations of theft; the idea here is that all human existence is based on taking from heaven. Heaven provides all things in the universe. The Chinese believe that our bodies are on loan and that after death our spirit returns to heaven and our body is broken down into its base elements to create other things. The whole idea of human existence is based on total support from heaven, so putting yourself in the best position to gain from heaven is not a negative move but is just like waiting in position for your sustenance to arrive.

☯ **Stealing from heaven means being in the right place at the right time doing the right thing. You can take all you need from heaven, but heaven will withhold it if you are not living in the correct manner.**

FISHING FOR SUCCESS

Stealing from heaven is to find a river where the salmon are running and set traps in it instead of fishing a dead river with a hook and no bait. It is making the minimum effort for the maximum reward. If you follow the Way with an honest heart and do not exploit others, then no matter what it is you need it will be there without your having to chase it. If you are struggling in life, rethinking your approach to the Way may set you on a more fruitful path.

PRESENCE AND ABSENCE

Behind the veil of reality lies absence, but what we think of as nothing is in fact everything.

The world is divided into what is there and what is not there:

- ***You*** **(有)** – presence (yang)
- ***Wu*** **(無)** – absence (yin)

Absence always carries the possibility of something that will be present in the future. For example, when a man and woman conceive a child they create a new combination of *chi* that was absent before. This is what is meant by the concept of *wu*. Conversely, presence is temporary and will lead to future absence. Yet again, yin is found in yang and yang is found in yin.

Before the movement of yinyang there was the absence of everything (*wu*), yet the possibility of everything becoming present (*you*). *You* and *wu* go hand in hand with yin and yang. Do not think in terms of a start point like the "big bang"; this is a continuous process. Things are created, they transform, they die, they return to become potential and the cycle continues.

☯ **Before the universe there was nothing but the Dao, and inside the Dao was the possibility for all things, then came time and the great machine of yinyang pumping *chi* around creation.**

THE EVER-CHANGING SKY

Take time to observe the sky and you will see you *and* wu *in action. A cloud has form and is observable* (you)*, while also holding the potential for future rain that does not currently exist* (wu)*.*

When the sky is clear and blue we know that it will not stay like that, and when clouds inevitably form we know that there will be a blue sky again sooner or later. The sky is always moving between you *and* wu.

THE THREE ASPECTS OF *WU*

The concept of wu *goes back to ancient ritual traditions and relates to female spirit-talkers. The following are three connected ideograms, all with different meanings yet all pronounced as* wu*:*

- Wu (無) – *absence*
- Wu (舞) – *dancing*
- Wu (巫) – *female spirit-talker*

In ancient days, wu *female spirit-talkers (巫) would perform* wu *dancing (舞) to the* wu *formless (無). In this context,* wu *(無) was the spirit world, home of heavenly deities known as* shen *(身). It was the place behind existence, the absence of matter. The task of the female spirit-talker was to bring existence from potential.*

THE 12 BLESSINGS AND CURSES

The 12 Blessings and Curses are positive and negative ways of viewing all situations that arise in life.

THE 12 BLESSINGS AND CURSES		
STAGE	BLESSING	CURSE
Birth	Vigour	Vulnerability
Bathing	Transformation	Instability
Dressing	Positive self-image	Vanity
Coming of age	Hard work	Life challenges
Peak condition	Tireless energy	Over-forcefulness
Ageing	Steadfastness	Aloofness
Sickness	Flexibility in mind	Unsettled status
Death	Unwavering mind	Coming to the end
In the tomb	Conservation	Hoarding
Energy collection	Unexpected benefits	Unexpected problems
Womb	Hope	Uncertainty
Awaiting rebirth	Cultivation	Effort and waiting

The stages should not be taken too literally. For example, the "death" stage does not necessarily mean an actual death; it may instead refer to the end of a situation such as a job or a relationship. In such a case, the benefit is that you know with an unwavering mind that you have to make a change; the curse is regret for something in your life that is coming to an end. All of the stages work in the same way, as metaphors for your life situation.

☯ Everything in life can be considered as either a blessing or a curse.

THE ULTIMATE VOID AND THE GREAT ULTIMATE

Before the reality of the universe there was the Ultimate Void (*wuji*). This was not nothing; it was something that did not yet exist. This was ultimate potential, the state of existence before the concept of existence. No laws of nature, no space, no time and not even the idea of "nothing". Then came the Great Ultimate (*taiji*), the force, fabric, thought, spark, singularity and laws of nature in the universe. This, as we have seen, is what created movement between yin and yang and generated *chi*.

People often find the idea of limitless non-existence represented by *wuji* difficult to understand. Think of it like this: inside the universe is both "something" and "nothing". It is like an empty room. There are walls (something) and an empty space (nothing). Without the something (the room), the nothing (the empty space) cannot exist. However, while the room is empty now, one day it will have an oak table in it. That table will be made from the wood of a tree that does not even exist yet. We know an acorn will come and from that a tree and from that a table. The acorn is not in a state of nothingness, it is in a state of potential. It is beyond creation and has yet to manifest.

☯ Everything we need in life is there in the Ultimate Void. We just have to follow the correct path and it will manifest.

DEVELOPING OUR SKILLS

Even though all we need is found in the realm of potential (the Ultimate Void), we still need to have the skills to manipulate the world in our favour.

The Chinese ideogram *shu* (術) represents the concept of ability and skills. This is perhaps better known in its Japanese form, *jutsu*, as in for example:

- ***Jujutsu* (柔術)** – grappling
- ***Kenjutsu* (剣術)** – swordsmanship
- ***Shinobi no jutsu* (忍術)** – the skills of the saboteur-spy

The term *shu* can be applied to any subject: skills in medicine, skills in yinyang, skills in pottery and so on. The following are historical Chinese terms that use the idea of *shu*:

- ***Wu shu* (武術)** – martial skills
- ***Xue shu* (學術)** – skills of the academic
- ***Ren shu* (仁術)** – skills of Confucianism
- ***Fa shu* (法術)** – skills of laws and codes
- ***Dao shu* (道術)** – skills of the Way
- ***Xin shu* (心術)** – skills of the mind

Shu (術) can also go beyond practical skills and be used to refer to semi-magical or spiritual activities requiring a particularly intense, zen-like focus. This can be seen in such fields as flower arranging, tea ceremonies and the martial arts.

☯ **Without ability there is no success. Dedicating ourselves to developing the skills we need is an important part of following the Way.**

PATHWAY TO PROGRESS

To benefit from the world, understand the following progression:

1. *The Way exists (*Dao*).*
2. *There is a need for skills (*shu*).*
3. *Do not engage with insignificant things.*
4. *Engage with things that matter.*
5. *Transform skill into benefit.*
6. *Live a clean and abundant life.*

STAYING IN THE CENTRE

Wuwei (無爲) is the idea of not forcing things to happen by pushing too hard in your desired direction. The two ideograms mean "absence" and "actions", so *wuwei* can be translated as "the absence of action". However, be careful not to misunderstand this as "do nothing". You still need to have a goal and work toward it.

Wuwei can also be thought of as remaining in the "centre of the circle", which means to engage with what life presents to you without forcing yourself to the edge of the position you are in.

Trust in heaven to take you where you need to go and provide you with the lessons you need to advance your spiritual being. All you have to do is follow the correct path. Do not rush ahead or retreat, do not try to avoid anything that is on the path. Stay focused on your goal and accept the challenges you need to face to get there.

There is an old Chinese teaching which states:

> *"True skill (*shu*) is the ability to stay in the centre without forcing anything to happen (*wuwei*) so that any deliberate actions you take (*youwei*, see below) are in response to what has happened."*

To follow the way of yinyang means leading life at a measured pace, using your skills to overcome any challenges that may arise but without deviating from the path.

☯ ***Wuwei* is to flow with day-to-day events while maintaining an overall goal. It means seeing situations arise, dealing with them positively and efficiently and then moving on.**

DIRECTED AND NON-DIRECTED ACTION

The opposite to *wuwei* (無爲) (non-directed and responsive action) is *youwei* (有爲) (directed action). *Youwei* is the closest to what people tend to do today to achieve their goals. They fix their mind on something, look at how to get what they want and make a grab for it. This is action specifically directed toward achieving a goal.

When people think *wuwei* means to do nothing, they could not be more wrong. To do nothing is actually to do something. For example, if you sit on a bench and wait for food to turn up, you are making a conscious decision. At the same time the universe is thinking, "I placed a shop just on the corner and gave you a job to earn money, so buy some food." This is *youwei* disguised as *wuwei*. In contrast, *wuwei* is to move about your day, positioning yourself in the best place, whether that be on the sunny side of a field to grow crops or in the most appropriate company for the job you want. *Wuwei* is doing what needs to be done for life to continue but not forcing the situation. It means waiting for opportunities to open up after you have found the correct position.

☯ ***Youwei* is to take actions specifically designed to achieve a certain goal. *Wuwei* is to put yourself in the right place and then deal with what happens.**

TWO WAYS OF LIVING IN SOCIETY

Youwei *and* wuwei *can also describe two contrasting approaches to living within society:*

- **Youwei** (有爲) *– to follow social norms and cultural rules*
- **Wuwei** (無爲) *– to move away from social convention and received opinions and eradicate social conditioning*

The path of society and the path of the Way do not always lead in the same direction.

ACTION AND INACTION

The concepts of *youshi* and *wushi* appear similar to *youwei* and *wuwei* on first inspection, but they are not the same and they must not be mixed up. The following table will make the distinction clear.

CHINESE CONCEPTS OF ACTION				
IDEOGRAM	CHINESE	JAPANESE	TRANSLATION	MEANING
有事	*Youshi*	*Yuji*	Action	To do tasks – be busy
無事	*Wushi*	*Buji*	Inaction	To do nothing – be lazy
有爲	*Youwei*	*Ui*	Directed action	To pursue goals
無爲	*Wuwei*	*Mui*	Responsive action	To live life naturally

Never confuse *wushi* (無事) and *wuwei* (無爲). *Wushi* is to do nothing, to laze around on the sofa with no goals, while *wuwei* is to engage with the world as it naturally occurs to you without pushing in a specific direction.

A person can act correctly in one of two ways:

- Spontaneous action in response to the world around them (*wuwei*)
- Direct and organized action within a social structure (*youwei*)

You can put yourself in the best position and react naturally or you can actively pursue your ambitions until they become a reality. The first way is to flow with the universe; the second is often to fight against it.

This leads to the following options:

- Let life happen naturally and aim to just exist in happiness (*wuwei*).

- Let life happen naturally and move into action when opportunities arise (*wuwei* with *youwei*).

- Push life in the direction you want and try to force the world and people around you to conform to your wishes (*youwei* with *youshi*).

- Have no dreams, no goals, no focus and do nothing (*wushi*).

☯ **Action (*youshi*) can be carried out in pursuit of ambitions (*youwei*) or as a natural response to life's events (*wuwei*). Inaction (*wushi*) is simple laziness.**

SKILLS OF THE WAY

The concept of *shu* was previously defined as skills within a certain area. Therefore, *Dao shu* (道術) means "skills (術) of the Way (道)". This means to have a deep understanding of the Dao and yinyang and to live life to the full by going with the flow of *wuwei* (not pushing against the situation) and to put yourself in position to "steal" (盜) from the Dao. *Dao shu* can be broken down into the following three subsections.

LIVE SIMPLY

Remove all unnecessary complications from your life. Focus on food, shelter and warmth and be grateful for these three simple pleasures. Avoid complex situations and let life flow freely.

When interacting with the world remember the teaching of the tree. A tree has hundreds of branches, thousands of twigs and uncountable leaves, yet it only has one root and trunk system. Therefore, in all your actions and interactions, search for the root of the issue; do not get tangled up in the leaves and branches.

☯ **Warmth and good cheer before hoarded gold. Root causes before insignificant details.**

GO WITH THE FLOW

In an old Chinese story, there was once a mighty waterfall that crashed down into a furiously swirling pool. The currents were so strong that no fish could live there. However, one man used to bathe in the violent waters every day and it appeared that he was having fun. When he was asked how he survived such strong currents, he said that he simply let them take him where they wanted, they swirled him around and took him for a jolly ride. He never struggled, because he knew that if he did he would soon become exhausted and drown. Having full trust in the Way, he floated along with it.

To our modern logical minds this sounds like stupidity; the water could pull the man under and kill him at any moment and it is folly to risk death like that. However, the point is to trust in the Way. A true master of the Dao has unshakeable faith in the Way to take them in the right direction. When the water pulls the man under, he does not fight it and become trapped; instead he allows the water to take him and then spit him out further downstream.

In the face of danger most people find it almost impossible to keep faith in the Way. Their logical mind kicks in, they start to strain against the situation and they go against the Way, which often leads to their downfall.

☯ **If we are true to the Dao and we relax and allow it to carry us along, it will take us to safety no matter how threatening the rocks and whirlpools of life appear.**

FOCUS ON THE INTERNAL

Human relationships – which in old China were ruled by schools of thought such as Confucianism – are complex. Engaging in society directly often leads to difficulties. Daoism teaches that if we truly understand the Way and the inner workings of our mind then we will automatically behave in the correct way and be able to identify any issues, no matter how complex the society in which we live.

☯ **Looking inside ourselves enables us to understand how the outside world works.**

FOLLOWING THE WAY OR FOLLOWING THE RULES

In this section we will examine the two contrasting concepts of *daode* (道德), which represents innate virtue and connection to the Dao, and *lunli* (倫理), which represents correct human relationships.

DAODE

This term consists of the *Dao* (道), "the Way", and *de* (德), "virtue". Together the two ideograms represent "the power/virtue of following the Way". This implies a harmonization with the Way and a skill in proper reaction rather than forced action. It is to innately know what is correct to do at the correct time rather than looking to external rules of morality for guidance. Each situation is different and to try to follow rules of morality is to become tangled in a web of confusion over what is and what is not correct.

LUNLI

Lun (倫) means "human relationships" and *li* (理) means "principles". Together they form a concept that means "the principles of human relationships". While many modern Chinese see *daode* and *lunli* as similar, they are, in fact, quite different. *Lunli* is about navigating the complex relationships and moral codes of society and so is more suited to Confucianism than to Daoism. It is based on a network of strict rules of conduct with little or no room for spontaneity.

☯ ***Daode* means to approach each situation with an innate feel for right and wrong in accordance with the Way, whereas *lunli* is to follow a defined set of responses to social situations.**

EMOTIONAL SKILLS

Xinshu (心術) means "the skill of emotions". The ideograms are *xin* (心), "heart", and *shu* (術), "skills". Fundamentally, it is about the proper use of emotion and being able to achieve a relaxed and flowing mental state.

One ancient scholar said that it is best not to try to run like a horse or fly like a bird, meaning that if you compare yourself unfavourably to others or attempt things that are not within your nature you will cause your mental state to become unbalanced. This does not mean you should have no emotions, but you should develop a calm outlook. If you burn with passion or anger you will become unsettled, so it is best to detach yourself from such strong emotions. Let your feelings come and go in gently rhythmic waves rather than crash into your consciousness in violent surges.

Confucianism also teaches its followers to control their emotions, but it advocates emotional restraint, whereas *xinshu* is to maintain a steady flow of feelings with no peaks or troughs. In the context of yinyang, *xinshu* is also concerned with maintaining a balance of *chi* energy to avoid surges in either yin or yang energy.

☯ ***Xinshu* is about settling the waters of the mind and balancing our emotions – we can still react to situations but we should not overreact.**

WHEN ALL ELSE FAILS

We have learned in this chapter the importance of being in the right place at the right time and using our skills to make the most of the opportunities that come our way. However, there may be occasions when we find ourselves in the wrong place at the wrong time and lacking in the skills that would help us in a particular situation. When this happens we need to fall back on our *yin* (因), which is "that on which to rely" – our basic ability to survive. Although this sounds exactly the same as the yin (陰) of yinyang, it is a completely different concept.

As an example, imagine that you need to cross a wide river. If you had been true to yinyang you would have waited until high summer when the river was low and easy to cross, but on this occasion your timing is off and you have arrived in a flood. If you had the necessary skills, this would be an opportunity to build a boat or a raft. Unfortunately, you do not have these skills. Therefore, all you have left to rely on is your *yin* (因), or natural ability. You will have to swim across the river and "fight" the water to get where you need to be, rather than going with the flow. This is not an ideal situation, but sometimes it cannot be helped.

☯ To avoid having to rely on our basic survival skills, we should focus on correct opportunity and timing and on developing the skills needed to take opportunities.

BODY, SPIRIT AND LIFE

The concepts *shen* (身), meaning "body", *shen* (神), meaning "spirit", and *sheng* (生), meaning "life", not only sound similar (or even identical) but are interrelated. *Shen* (身) is a body that is animated with life, not to be confused with *shen* (神), which is the spirit that inhabits the body and divides in two after death, while *sheng* is the concept of life itself. The concepts are connected in that keeping your body (as well as your mind and emotions) as healthy as possible nourishes the spirit and is associated with a good life. Body, spirit and life are one.

☯ A body has life within it and life is to be enjoyed, but inside the body is the spirit which, upon death, when all the *chi* has been spent, will depart and divide into yin and yang.

THE FIVE FOCUSES OF SAGEHOOD

Now understanding that *shen* (身) means "body", there are five basic ideas connected to the body that, if followed, will lead to sagehood.

- ***Ashen* (安身)** – to have peace within the body and mind (do not overcomplicate your life with trivial things, keep things simple and avoid overstressing your body and mind)

- ***Shoushen* (守身)** – to guard the body (pay attention to your own body and look out for signs of damage, wear and tear, and stress)

- ***Guishen* (貴身)** – to value the body (eat well, keep clean both internally and externally, and remember your responsibility to do what you can to maintain your health)

- ***Fanshen* (返身)** – to look back on your past – literally, "body-return" (understand that your body will change and that it may not do what it once could do, only push your body to its current limits and do not measure yourself against past achievements)

- ***Xiushen* (修身)** – to cultivate the body (perfect your body, build the shape you want and put effort into your appearance)

Sages are renowned for cultivating their minds, but they also know the importance of cultivating the body.

THE SAGE AND THE SCHOLAR

In Chinese culture and folklore you will sometimes see a battle between the broad-minded sage and the narrow-minded scholar. In this battle, scholars tend to see the world only from the perspective of their specialism, whereas sages tend to look at the world as a whole and produce a better society.

SPIRITUAL ILLUMINATION

When a human is working in perfect order and has reached sagehood, they are said to have achieved *shenming* (神明), "illumination". The ideograms are "spirit" (神) and "bright" (明), giving a literal meaning of "bright spirit", which also has a deeper significance. The *chi* of the body is absorbed from the world around as the sage practises perfect yinyang, but *chi* also radiates out from them because of their inner clarity. Therefore, to have *shenming* is to "steal" from the universe in full and to burn with the power of creation by leading a pure life. *Chi* flows around you, *chi* flows within you and *chi* flows from you when you perfectly follow the Way.

☯ **The Chinese ideograms for "spirit" (神) and "bright" (明) illustrate how a human can become illuminated by following ancient ways laid down by sages of the past.**

MENTAL ATTITUDES AND EMOTION

When approaching the mind, there are five mental attitudes to consider as well as six basic emotions. Both sets must be considered when thinking about personal growth.

The five mental attitudes are:

- ***Ren*** **(仁)** – benevolence
- ***Yi*** **(義)** – righteousness
- ***Li*** **(禮)** – ritual
- ***Zhi*** **(智)** – wisdom
- ***Xin*** **(信)** – trust

The six emotions are:

- ***Xi*** **(喜)** – happiness
- ***Nu*** **(怒)** – anger
- ***Ai*** **(哀)** – sadness
- ***Le*** **(樂)** – joy
- ***Ai*** **(愛)** – love
- ***Tan*** **(貪)** – greed

If there is an imbalance between the emotions, then the *chi* of the body will be disrupted and illness will manifest.

☯ **Maintaining a calm mind is part of maintaining healthy *chi* and a calm mind is achieved through proper mental attitude.**

THE WAY OF HUMANS

The way of water is to manage water to meet our needs while understanding its natural "flow". For example, if we build a dam or create a seal we know that water will want to find a way through it. Another approach might be to divert the water so that it can continue to flow.

The way of humans is like this. It is not to create barriers or complications but to find a way to work within the natural flow of human properties, to take the path of least resistance toward perfection. However, finding an easier path is not the same as doing nothing.

Everything has a way – the way of tea, the way of horses, the way of fishing, and so on – and each one uses high-level skills to achieve the maximum benefit. The way of humans is just another way to master.

With its suppression of emotion, Confucianism creates a metaphorical dam within humans to minimize conflict, whereas yinyang theory is to have humans flow naturally like water and harmonize together.

MASTERING MIND AND BODY BEFORE MASTERING OTHERS

If a leader does not have mastery over their own body and mind, then they cannot attempt to steer the affairs of the world without causing chaos to erupt. A healthy body is trim, flexible and regulated, while a healthy mind is clear and free from corruption and greed. Only when a person has mastered the ability to maintain a healthy and pure self can they focus on fixing problems in the wider world.

Before forcing others to follow their way, a leader needs to consider whether they have mastered the Way.

REWARD AND PUNISHMENT

Society is based on reward and punishment. Traditionally, reward should be given without delay and be slightly more than is justified for the action that earned it; while punishment should be slightly less severe than the offence that earned it and should not be carried out in haste but should be done only after serious deliberation.

- Reward is of the element of yang.
- Punishment is of the element of yin.

If there is too much punishment in society or too much reward then the bonds of control and harmony will collapse. Excessive punishment will result in rebellions and riots, while excessive reward will result in degeneration.

Reward and punishment in society should be balanced like yin and yang.

HUMANS AND THE UNIVERSE

There are many branches of Daoism and many aspects to its philosophy, but it has settled into a set of teachings that have come together from the first oracle bones of the ancient past all the way through to the Palace Edition of the I-Ching and beyond. This way of living within the Way and yinyang has set the background for Chinese thought for most of its existence. These historical teachings are summarized in the following lists as a guideline for you to understand your position in the world and universe beyond.

HUMAN EXISTENCE IS A PRACTICAL EXPERIENCE

- Practical human existence must come before abstract philosophical ideas.

- Human existence is subjective and people's minds will project what they believe onto the outside world.

- Humans can think in abstract thoughts and project ideas about the future.

- Humans naturally reflect on their own experience.

- Humans can make changes to make their future better.

HUMANS CHANGE

- Changes in nature come from the Dao and human experience.

- Humans observe the flow of reality and start to see patterns of change.

- The differences between individual humans come from the Dao, which divides into all things and gives all things individuality.

POSITIONING HUMANS WITHIN THE WORLD

- The world is a system that continues to produce the things humans need.

- Humans should position themselves within the landscape to benefit from the natural abundance of the world.

- The world will continue to produce as long as balance within it is maintained.

- Forcing nature the wrong way or constructing social barriers and systems is to move away from the natural order.

THE UNITY OF HUMANKIND

- Harmony is actually found in opposites: men and women, sun and moon, dark and light, and so on. Differences make for overall balance.

- Harmony is a state of balance between opposites that leads to a vibrant existence.

- Humans can unite in the understanding that opposites are the key to reality and that it is best to see the whole picture rather than focus on any differences.

Life started before matter, the "mind" of the Dao or universal principle brought reality into being and all of reality started as a single principle. From there, it divided into and created all things and the whole point of existence is to experience the oppositeness of everything, from sun and shadow on a mountainside to the differences between male and female.

All aspects of society are based on relationships between people who are different. We should be happy to meet people who are not the same as ourselves and then find a harmonious balance within nature.

There is abundance in the world if humans learn how to get the most from the planet naturally and equitably, but to artificially force the earth will cause problems.

Social and political barriers create enmity and make us forget that we are here to celebrate difference not to hate it. Humans should strive for diversity without restricting others and create a future where people are happy in their own worlds and do not dream of taking from others. Humans should live in their own private paradise where the world provides for them without a struggle because they have positioned themselves correctly. The Dao provides for all but will kill if humans try to corrupt it or stray into the wrong area at the wrong time.

☯ **The world is a place for humans to manipulate to create abundance for a pleasurable existence. However, overpopulation, uncontrolled technological advances and putting profit first can lead to a hellish imbalance within yinyang.**

A MOVE TOWARD THE ANDROGYNOUS

The aim of the human is to move toward a stronger balance of yin and yang and toward a lesser difference between men and women. It is best to be careful here and not overlay modern gender issues on this ancient thought. It is not for men to become less masculine or women to become less feminine, but men should maintain a strong basis of yang energy and build up yin power and women should maintain a strong yin element while building up yang. This is not about clothes, gestures or societal roles; it is about both sexes strengthening and balancing their internal energy so that men are not brutish and women are not passive. Both should work in harmony and balance, remembering their gender but combining both sides of yinyang in the quest for perfection.

☯ **Women should be stronger in yin but hold on to yang, while men should be stronger in yang but maintain yin. Together, they should maintain a correct overall balance of yin and yang.**

ACHIEVING TRANSCENDENCE

Humans must transcend their base needs in order to attain perfection. The human mind is full of confusion, but once you have fully understood yinyang you will engage in actions that are not forced, which will lead to a quiet mind in a pure and healthy body. Such a union is divine (*shen*), and if a person reaches this state of divinity that person becomes a dragon.

Those who perfectly understand yinyang and live accordingly can attain transcendence.

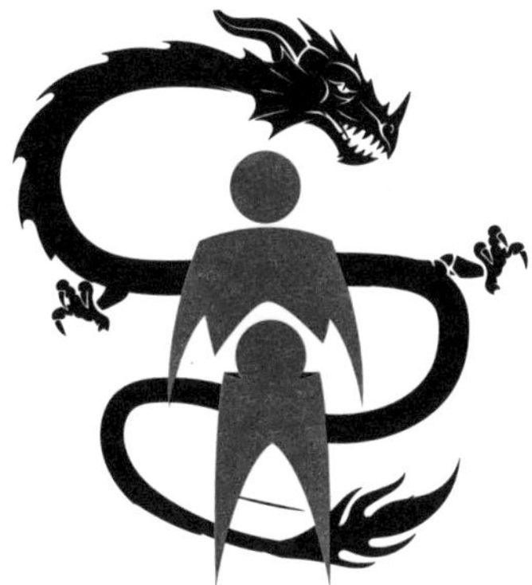

ABOVE: The dragon is the image of human mental perfection.

THE DRAGON

In Daoist stories and fables the dragon often features as a symbol of the transcended spirit, the ultimate state before perfection is achieved. A spirit such as this is formidable and stands alone as a beacon of strength. This is why Lao Tzu is often known as the Dragon.

THE PERFECT HUMAN

The idea of the perfect human, the ultimate goal in most Chinese schools of thought, is represented by various ideograms, which can be translated as "true gentleman", "honest human", "genuine person", "utmost person", "sage", "master", and so on. They all denote a person who has taken full control of their internal functions and accumulated enough wisdom to enable them to engage perfectly with all situations, fully understand the heavens and the earth and live a pure, full life.

The perfect human follows yinyang, harmonizes with yinyang and masters yinyang.

THE WATER MIND

Ideograms associated with water are often used by the Chinese and Japanese to represent the levelling out of the mind and the control of the emotions. Like water, the mind may be turbulent, but when the disturbance has passed, both water and mind find their own level and become calm. Calm water reflects, and so does a calm mind.

THE PERFECT LIFE

Some people are tempted to study ancient Chinese wisdom, especially Daoism, because they think that it will lead them to immortality. However, the Chinese long ago gave up on the idea of the elixir of life and alchemical Daoism. Instead they look to achieve a different kind of immortality by merging with the Dao so that after death their spirit will live within the Dao and not dissipate.

Our task in following yinyang is not to extend our life, but to find the perfect position in which to live with meaning. We must put ourselves where we can communicate and integrate with the Dao and engage with what the universe presents at all times.

☯ **We should not overstay our welcome, but neither should we waste the time we have.**

COMMUNICATING WITH THE DAO

To maintain the perfect life you should follow these guidelines:

- Have faith in the Dao.
- Look after your body and mind.
- Position yourself in the physical world and in society where you will be happy.
- Do not let greed lead you into the wrong position.

- Understand that true wealth is found in a healthy and productive life surrounded by people you love and who love you.
- Live life to the full and engage with it.
- Focus on preserving and maintaining a high level of energy.
- Continue to observe yinyang in nature.
- Do not regret having to die.
- Know that when you die you will join with the Dao.

☯ **Remember, warmth and good cheer before hoarded gold.**

WORKING WITH YINYANG:

Act in accordance with the Dao

You are at the centre of your world and your relationship to the Dao is all that matters. This is the same for everyone, and the secret to the universe is just this. If everyone focuses on their own path toward the Dao, without unbalancing society or earth's natural resources, then we will all live in harmony, want for nothing and paradise will be achieved. It is the search for more that leads humankind to function imperfectly; it is our own misgivings that cause our troubles. Be in the right place at the right time, take only what you need and know when you have enough. Heaven is watching you, the moon and stars see all things and make all things right in the end, but only you can tread the path of the Dao.

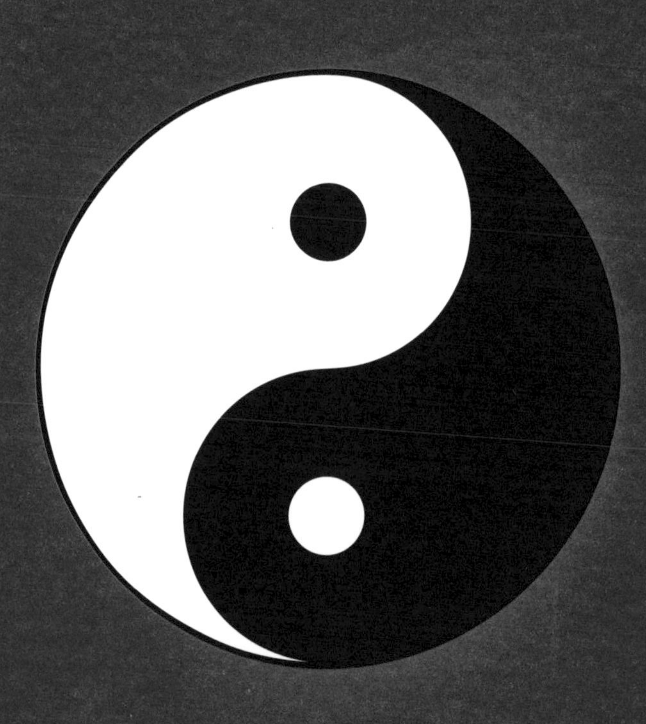

A QUICK GUIDE TO YINYANG

A QUICK GUIDE TO YINYANG

Having digested the whole text now, and having started on your inner journey toward the Dao and to the use of yinyang, you can use the following series of bullet points and lists to help remember the process and live a life in tune with nature. Return to these lists to keep your understanding in shape and your actions in alignment with yinyang.

THE UNIVERSE, YINYANG AND THE WAY

- Often translated as the Way, the Dao means the pathways and laws behind existence.
- The Dao is the pattern of the universe, it is the laws of nature behind the visible world.
- Yinyang was at the beginning of the universe, and it will be there at the end.
- Yinyang movement is the basis for all creation.
- Yinyang is about harmonizing with the Way.
- You do not need to look for the beginning of the universe nor the end; simply exist in its river flowing through time.
- The movement of the primordial fabric of the universe creates both yin and yang and *chi*.
- The Dao is unchanging but the universe is always in flux.
- Consciousness and matter need each other to exist.
- No one knows if the Dao is conscious of humans. However, we have to be in tune with the Dao to benefit from it.

- There is more than one story of how the universe was created and not all of them involve yin and yang.
- One theory of the origin of the universe is that it came from an egg that was broken open by a great being.
- The classical theory of the origin of the universe is that the Dao moved into yin and yang and that sparked the *chi* energy of the universe and from this came all life in all of its forms.
- There was a stage before the universe divided into yin and yang, a pre-yinyang state where the possibility for division existed.
- The question of when time started creates problems for modern people.
- Neo-Confucianists understand the Daoist idea of the Dao (道) but may instead use the term *li* (理), which means "the principle".
- The Way (with a capital letter) means the laws behind the universe; the way (with a small letter) means a specific path taken by a human toward perfection. For example, the "way of heaven" is a mixture of astronomy and astrology.
- The ideogram for the Way can be taken to represent either a person walking down a path or just the path itself.
- In Buddhism the Way means to follow the teachings of Buddha and gain enlightenment.
- Some texts say that the Dao is neither good nor bad. However, many teachings maintain that good action is preferred by the innate laws of the universe.
- Heaven supplies all things for humans, from the sun to the crops, from the fish in the sea to the raw materials for tools. All humans are given bounty by heaven.

- There are only two states in the universe: that which is in existence (known as *you*) and that which is in a state of potential (known as *wu*).
- The Ultimate Void (*wuji*) is the pre-universe, while the Great Ultimate (*taiji*) is the universe in movement, the spark of the universe, the essence of yin and yang before separation.

YINYANG BASICS

- Yinyang is the matrix of creation.
- Yinyang is a single term made up of two parts. When you are referring to the concept as a whole, use the single word yinyang; when you are referring to the two elements individually, divide the term into yin and yang.
- There are different Chinese ways of saying "yinyang" and the western pronunciation is only an approximation of these.
- Just because two things are yin or yang, it does not make them the same – it is simply a categorization. All of existence is either yin or yang, but there are countless things in the world.
- Yin energy brings things into form, while yang gives them their nature.
- Yin and yang is the study of real-world phenomena, such as stars, the wind, the rain and so on.
- Heaven, humans and the earth are in a vertical relationship.
- All things living on the earth are in a horizontal relationship.
- Certain elements, such as the Five Phases (wood, fire, earth, metal, water), interact with each other in a circular relationship.

- Yin and yang are constantly flowing in and out of dominance and subservience. Overall there is balance but that does not mean a steady line of neutrality.

- Whether something is yin or yang depends on the context it is being viewed in.

- Yin and yang do not try to destroy each other; they simply move in and out of dominance. There is no war between them and there never has been.

- Yin and yang only exist in relation to each other.

- When talking about yin and yang, "negative" is used in a scientific way, as in the negative pole of a magnet or the negative terminal of a battery. It does not mean "bad".

- Yinyang is like the roots of a tree: you cannot see them but they give life.

- Yinyang cannot be described directly; it is only done through analogy.

- Yinyang is about contrasting elements coming together to make something that will function well in the world – like a wheel that combines hard wood for strength and soft wood for flexibility.

- Yinyang is a single entity with two polar opposites and a spectrum in between.

- Yin is found inside of yang and yang inside of yin.

- No matter whether yin or yang is in power, know that the weaker one is contained within the stronger and is waiting for its turn to rise.

- The yinyang symbol is called the *taiji*.

- The dots of opposite colour in each half of the *taiji* represent the presence of yin and yang within their opposites, showing that all things move in a cycle.

- Sometimes what you need is the solid yang aspect of an object, like the blade of a spade; at other times you need the yin space inside an object, like that within an empty jug. The usefulness of an object may be either its yang or its yin aspect.

- The Five Phases each cycle through a state of yin and a state of yang, making 10 "branches" overall. These are called the 10 Heavenly Stems.

- Just because something has no form does not mean that it has no effect. Think of electricity.

- Things either change their form, such as rock into sand, or reproduce so that their line continues down the ages, such as animals and plants.

- Living things have a creation point, an existence, a decay stage, a point of death and a period of dissolution.

- There are two types of harmony: constructed harmony, where individual parts fit perfectly together but can be separated; and blended harmony, where the ingredients once mixed together are no longer identifiable individually.

- There are three types of yin (greater yin, lesser yin and declining yin) and three types of yang (greater yang, lesser yang and bright yang), allowing the possibility of many different combinations.

- Timing in yinyang does not mean counting hours; it means correct action in the appropriate situation.

- Yang is strong in the short term but will die and allow yin to return to dominance.

- Each season and direction has different strengths of *chi* at different times of the year. There are tables included in this book to work each one out (see pages 183).

- When a living being dies, yin *chi* moves downward to the ground and yang *chi* floats up to the sky.

- Human *chi* has an effect on the balance of yin and yang *chi* in the surrounding area.

THE LANDSCAPE

- South is normally at the top of an ancient map (from the northern hemisphere) because people looked up to the sun and the sun passes to the south.

- If you face the sun then it rises on your left and sets on your right.

- The summer solstice is full yang and the start of yin, while the winter solstice is full yin and the start of yang.

- The world can be divided into six directions: north, south, east, west, up and down. Alternatively, from the point of view of a human: ahead, behind, left, right, above and below.

- The earth is considered as a square because of the angles on the ground while the sky is considered as round because it is a dome.

- Day and night is a process of yin moving into yang and yang moving into yin.

- Sometimes the translation of colours within the natural world from one language to another is difficult because often ancient languages are talking about the colours they see in the environment around them, not artificial colours created by humans.

- There are two ways in which yin and yang are associated with directions. Be careful not to mix the two systems up. The first version says that east and south are yang; the second version says that south and north are yang.

- There are 12 basic directions set 30 degrees apart on the horizon of the earth and each one is represented by an animal. The centre points of each direction are as follows:
    - Rat 0°
    - Ox 30°
    - Tiger 60°
    - Hare 90°
    - Dragon 120°
    - Snake 150°
    - Horse 180°
    - Ram 210°
    - Monkey 240°
    - Cockerel 270°
    - Dog 300°
    - Boar 330°

- The parts of a river are divided into yin and yang, even though the river itself is of water and is fundamentally yin.

- When the tide of the sea is fully in and at full power, it is at full yin, but when it is out it is at full yang. This is the opposite of what you would expect given that yang is normally seen as "full". However, because water is yin a tide at full height is associated with total yin.

- The purpose of *feng shui* is to collect *chi* and keep it close to your home.

- According to *feng shui*:
    - Your home should face south.
    - You should have a water source to the front.
    - You should have mountains or hills to the rear.
    - Splashing water scatters *chi*.

- The south is yang and the north is yin. However, when it comes to the banks of rivers the opposite is true because the north bank of a river faces south and the south bank faces north.

YINYANG IN HISTORY

- Yinyang started as the observation of visible natural phenomena and developed into theories about the unseen properties of *chi*.
- The school of yinyang was called the House of Yin and Yang but its teachings were lost and now all we have are reconstructed selections from its curriculum.
- The school of yinyang was very varied in its teachings, ranging from the study of the stars to the interpretation of dreams, from understanding the parts of the face to complex sex rituals.
- Even though yinyang was around at the start of Chinese history, it may have been codified by members of the Confucian class of gentlemen who had enough money to be able to spend time studying. However, this does not account for the lay magic users and other spiritual teachers who also made a study of yinyang.
- A nine-square grid represents a mixture of yin and yang. Yin because everything square is yin and yang because nine, the highest number in yinyang, is yang.
- The famous yinyang symbol known as the *taiji* was invented long after the idea of yinyang was established.
- The origin of the *taiji* is not known for certain. It could have been adopted from the Romans, it could represent two rivers merging or it could depict the path of the sun and the moon in orbit.
- There were other ways to illustrate the idea of yinyang before the *taiji* was invented.

- In old days there were diagrams that mapped out how the universe worked. They can often be read two ways: from creation to destruction and from destruction to the original source of all life.
- Lao Tzu, the famous author of the Dao De Jing, said that the Way cannot be named, that it is formless and that if you can grasp it then you are not talking about the real Way.
- Despite this, Lao Tzu is not saying that you should not attempt to understand and describe the Way. People often misunderstand this point, but his entire book is about trying to understand the Way.
- Nowadays the concept of "heaven, earth and man" should be translated as "heaven, earth and humans". In the past "man" stood for both male and female.
- There are three basic sets of elements from the ancient world: the Greek, the Indian and the Chinese. There may originally have been some form of connection between them but if so it has long been lost. Consider them as separate and know that in this book we are dealing with the five Chinese elements, which are what we refer to as the Five Phases.
- Some Daoist masters tried to find the secret of immortality by studying alchemy. Having failed in this quest, many turned to the idea of internal alchemy and the pursuit of the immortality of the spirit.
- Yinyang is one of the four main pillars of Asian warfare.
- It is said that some Chinese stringed instruments represent yin and yang.
- Music conveys emotion from one human to another. It can sway the feeling of a whole crowd of people.
- Music is yang while dance (including ritual dance) is yin. Others say that music is a combination of yin and yang.

- Legend says that dance was invented to regulate yin and yang energy in the body and the cosmos.

ANCIENT CHINA

- The ancient peoples of what we now call China were of various ethnicities. The unification of China is a later development than yinyang.
- Chinese civilization is said to have started with the legendary Yellow Emperor, who is associated with the earth element.
- In old Chinese the term "ten thousand things" means "all things", "multitudes" or "all creation".
- The Chinese political structure is based on yinyang.
- Houses and even whole cities are built with *feng shui* and yinyang in mind.
- A grave is known as a "house of yin" and the principles of correct grave positioning were possibly the trigger for *feng shui*.
- The Chinese are believed to have created a system of eight directions based on a nine-square field layout with a shared well for farmers in the central square.
- The Asian calendar is different from the western version, which means that dates often do not match. Whenever you are told "x day of y month", remember that this refers to the Asian calendar, which starts counting from Chinese New Year.
- The Chinese have to adjust their traditional calendar every year to match their system to the movements of the moon around the earth and the earth around the sun.

- Each Chinese dynasty of the imperial age was associated with a colour that represented its connection to the Five Phases.

- Each dynasty of ancient China was associated with one of the Five Phases in the same sequence as the cycle of destruction, which reflects the idea that each dynasty took power from the one before it (although in actual history it was often more complicated than that).

- Tradition holds that an omen was given before each new Chinese dynasty came to power.

- In ancient China the horse and chariot was symbolic of the whole cosmos and the two human drivers represented yin and yang.

- A village or town can change the weather by engaging in either yin or yang activities.

- The Hundred Schools of Thought refers to a time in China when many ideas and schools of thought cemented into organizations with defined boundaries between them, each one looking to rule China correctly.

- Circular Chinese coins with a square hole in the middle represent yang and yin and heaven and earth. The circle represents heaven while the square hole represents earth. However, the circle of the coin is solid, unlike heaven, and the square is empty, unlike earth.

- Some masters will perform a ritual dance within a square to commemorate the workings and relationships of yinyang.

- In ancient China before the written word, objects such as bones or tortoise shells were burned and the resulting crack lines were observed for divination. These lines may have been the origin of the trigram and hexagram system used in the I-Ching manual.

- Water symbols were inscribed on buildings to protect against fire.

- Rituals were performed to the four cardinal points and the centre to honour the animal guardians of those directions.

- The traditional Chinese year is divided into 24 parts, all based on the seasonal and agricultural year. These are known as the 24 Solar Terms.

- The Chinese year is divided into four seasons of 72 days with 18 transition or earth days between each season, to give a total of 360 days. This meant that adjustments had to be made each year to keep the calendar correct.

- Original Chinese texts often contained an extra layer of wordplay or alliteration, which is usually lost in translation.

- Painters are yang because they move, while the subject to be painted is yin because it is still.

- Within a painting there are areas of yin and yang. The defined areas are yang and the implied areas are yin. There are also further sub-divisions such as dark and light, internal and external, and so on.

- The festival for the dead is on the fifteenth day of the seventh month in the Chinese calendar. The fifteenth day is always the day of a full moon because the calendar is based on observations of the moon. Remember that the moon is an aspect of yin and yin is an aspect of death.

- An altar in a yin direction is yin while one in a yang direction is yang, but within this general classification the left side of *any* altar is yang while the right side is yin.

- Marriages should take place in spring when yin and yang energies mix. However, the various schools of *feng shui* may add further calculations to this.

- Divination and omens are considered a significant part of yinyang theory. Do not dismiss them as superfluous.

- Divination can be done in many ways, including through stars, sticks, coins, shells and the human body.

- Palm reading and physiognomy are important parts of ancient Chinese culture but are also found in Greece.

THE I-CHING

- The I-Ching is a book of symbols known as hexagrams and includes commentaries on divination.
- I-Ching is pronounced "eee-Ching" or "yee-Ching", not "eye-Ching".
- A trigram has three lines and a hexagram has six lines. Each hexagram comprises two trigrams. There are eight trigrams, which can be combined to make a total of 64 hexagrams.
- Hexagrams are a representation of yinyang and the movement between yin and yang.
- The I-Ching has gone through many changes and been added to over the ages.
- The I-Ching is said to have been built in four stages by four people, but this is just a legend.
- In history there have been different versions of the I-Ching, but today there is a single unified version.
- The I-Ching is a manual to help humans make the correct changes in their lives.
- You should use the I-Ching to observe external changes in the world and understand changes within yourself.
- The trigrams and hexagrams of the I-Ching are made up of two basic types of line: yin lines, which are broken; and yang lines, which are solid. However, these two types of line are further subdivided into "young" and "old" lines.

- A hexagram can either be static, meaning that the divination result stays the same, or it can transform into a new version if it contains any transforming lines. This will only become apparent during the casting of a divination.
- When the lines of a hexagram transform, it simply means that a yin line changes to a yang line or vice versa.
- Only old lines transform; young lines stay as they are. For example, an old yang line becomes a young yin line when it transforms.
- Trigrams are either predominantly yin or predominantly yang. There are none with a true balance of both.
- Always look at the composition of trigrams and hexagrams. You may notice that yin and yang flow through in a progression.
- All books on the I-Ching should include a 64-hexagram table. Sometimes this is hidden away at the back of the book, so check carefully.
- The table of hexagrams may differ from book to book, but the numbers and matching hexagrams should always be the same.
- Hexagrams are built from the bottom up, so the first line you cast goes at the bottom and you keep casting until you get to the sixth line at the top.
- A hexagram can be divided into three pairs of lines. The top pair represents heaven; the middle pair, humans; the bottom pair, earth.
- Hexagrams are usually displayed as six lines one on top of the other, but can also be represented in other ways – for example, as three concentric circles.

THE FIVE PHASES

- The Five Phases (wood, fire, earth, metal, water) are the connection between the source of the universe and finished creation.
- The Five Phases represent types of energy, not physical elements.
- Before Five Phase theory became popular, the ancient Chinese saw fire and water as the building blocks of the world.
- Often you will see other translations such as "five elements", "five aspects", "five powers", and so on. In this book they have been translated as "five phases" to emphasize the fact that they move in cyclical relationships with each other.
- The Five Phases can represent the movement of attitudes in the mind and so can track human behaviour.
- Wood is in the east, its colour is light green-blue and it is guarded by a light green-blue dragon.
- Wood is connected to the directions of the Tiger, Hare and Dragon, which are all in the east quadrant.
- Wood is connected to spring.
- Fire is in the south, its colour is red and it is guarded by a giant red bird.
- Fire is connected to the directions of the Snake, Horse and Ram, which are all in the south quadrant.
- Fire is connected to summer.
- Metal is in the west, its colour is white and it is guarded by a white tiger.
- Metal is connected to the directions of the Monkey, Cockerel and Dog, which are all in the west quadrant.

- Metal is connected to autumn.
- Water is in the north, its colour is black and it is guarded by a black tortoise.
- Water is connected to the directions of the Boar, Rat and Ox, which are all in the north quadrant.
- Water is connected to winter.
- Earth is connected to the centre, its colour is gold and it is guarded by a golden dragon.
- Earth is often considered to represent a period of transition. It is connected to the inter-cardinal points and the transitional days between the four seasons.
- As well as being connected to the end of one season and the beginning of the next, earth is also particularly associated with late summer, when the yang half of the year gives way to yin. Always it represents a period of transition.
- An alternative version says that earth is connected to the directions of the Dragon, Ram, Dog and Ox.
- Sometimes the Five Phases are shown in cosmological order, with wood, earth and metal on a horizontal plane and fire, earth and water on a vertical plane. This reflects the way they exist in nature.
- Sometimes in the Five Phases you will see some of the phases described as mother and child or grandfather and grandchild and so on. These are ways to refer to relationships between specific phases.
- The Five Phases can work in two basic ways: the life cycle and the death cycle.
- The Five Phases have a counteracting cycle, which is the death cycle in reverse.

- There are variations on the classic Five Phases system featuring wood, fire, earth, metal and water but they have fallen out of fashion.

- Earth supports everything, fire gives heat, metal destroys things, water cools and wood is used to produce.

- Each of the Five Phases and yin and yang have numbers attached to them. The Five Phases are numbered in two cycles from one to 10 and yin and yang alternately from one to nine. However, the two numbering systems do not match.

- Impending disaster, whether inside the human body or in the world at large, can be signalled by a high degree of imbalance within the Five Phases.

- Earth is one of the Five Phases, but heaven is not. Some ancients believed that there were actually six true aspects, adding heaven to the classic five of earth, fire, metal, water and wood.

- The Five Phases can also represent the parts of civilized society: landscape management (wood), agriculture (earth), irrigation (water), power (fire) and tools (metal). If these are approached correctly human society will flourish.

- The Five Phases are aligned with the five virtues of Confucius (see page 241).

- To throw metal (yin) into water (yin) in honour of the dead (yin) is an act of reverence.

TRADITIONAL CHINESE MEDICINE

- Chinese medicine is about maintaining health. It favours preventative measures, or treatments applied when your body shows the very first signs of illness.

- If you overreact to an excess of yin or yang you can sometimes push things too far in the opposite direction.
- The human body is built to last 100 years, but each bad action takes some time off that total.
- Use coolness to calm heat.
- Purge "evil" toxins from the body.
- Strengthen the spleen and the stomach.
- The body contains *fu* (yang) organs and *zang* (yin) organs.
- The body has designated areas and organs of yin and yang.
- Each part can then be further divided into its yin and yang parts. Context and relationship are the key.
- The organs of the body are each associated with a certain emotion.
- If you experience an excess of a certain emotion, this will affect the organ associated with that emotion and may cause illness.
- Within the human body, the bones and flesh represent earth and soil, the eyes and ears represent the sun and moon, the top of the head represents the north star (Polaris), urine represents the waters of the world and the internal organs represent hills and valleys.
- The human body is divided into parts of heaven (moving aspects) and parts of earth (static aspects).
- Meridians are channels that carry *chi* throughout the body. Along each of these meridians are checkpoints or junctions commonly known as "acupuncture points".
- A central idea in Traditional Chinese Medicine is that each part of the body has a structure and a function.

- When observing a patient there is a series of checks to start with (see page 249–50).

- Traditional healing involves finding the root cause, which often cannot be seen. Many people try mistakenly to treat the manifestation and not the hidden cause.

- It can be difficult to tell whether yin or yang is the root cause of a problem. Sometimes treatment can require the opposite of what you expect.

- The basic rule is to treat heat with coolness and cold with warmth. However, there are situations where this principle does not apply or it is reversed.

- Do not treat a deficit of yin by reducing yang or a deficit of yang by reducing yin. What the patient needs is an increase in the aspect that is lacking.

- Similarly, do not add more yin or yang to a patient if what they need is a reduction in the other aspect.

- The pulse is very important in Traditional Chinese Medicine and it is measured in a different way from in the West. There are different categories of pulse and men and women also tend to have different types of pulse.

- *Shiatsu* practitioners work from the floor and stretch and meditate before the session.

- Too much yin or yang energy will result in over-powerful dreams and if these persist it will lead to ill health.

HUMANS AND LIFE

- The human "soul" is broken up into multiple parts that do different things and go to different places after death.

- Human relationships are a joining of yinyang.
- Positions within the family are dictated by yinyang.
- The dragon symbolizes the male or yang while the mare represents the female or yin.
- Yin and yang are associated with female and male in humans and other creatures, but they do not themselves have any gender.
- Yinyang does not put one gender above the other. Male and female are equal in the eyes of the Dao.
- Yang is superior to yin in human relationships, but this does not mean men are superior to women. In this context, the comparison is senior to junior and this is regardless of gender.
- Men contain feminine aspects and women contain masculine aspects but there should be an overall balance of yin and yang across the population.
- Stop thinking of yourself as being a tiny point on a map. Instead see yourself as the centre of the whole landscape.
- You see the universe as separate parts but the universe sees you as something which is a part of it.
- There is enough in the world for all people as long as we do not take too much. If you follow the Dao, the Dao will give you as much as you need (but maybe not as much as you want).
- The universe can give you what you need to live in comfort, for it is far more powerful than even the greatest worldly power. You just have to learn how to communicate with the Dao.
- Every form of movement provokes a reaction somewhere else. This applies to the physical, the spiritual and the relationship you have with heaven.

- Yin and yang can swing to extremes and when this happens humans usually suffer.

- Upon death, most people's souls divide into two parts: the yang part, which goes up to heaven; and the yin part, which stays on earth. However, according to some traditions, the souls of those who have lived a perfect life join with the Dao upon death; and the souls of those whose existence has been worthless break down completely.

- Sex represents the union of heaven and earth through human action.

- In sex, a man must steal yin energy from a woman by giving her as many orgasms as possible.

- A man's penis is called a "tool of yang" while a woman's vagina is called a "house of yin".

- Every situation can be viewed as either a blessing or a curse.

- Put simply, the concept of *shu* is to have ability in a certain field, but it also has connotations of a deeper ability within the Dao that can enable a human to progress to a higher level of existence.

- There are two ways to approach human interaction: to follow a complex set of social rules or to go with the flow and do what feels correct.

- *Shen* (身) means our body, not to be confused with the identically transliterated *shen* (神), which is the spirit that inhabits the body and divides in two after death. The similar term *sheng* (生) is the concept of life itself.

- The human mind is like a river – if you create a dam or blockage, problems will arise.

- Society needs a balance of reward and punishment. Too much either way and it will collapse.

USING YINYANG TO CREATE A BETTER LIFE

- If the whole world acted in the correct way, there would be heaven on earth.
- Success in terms of yinyang theory means to be in the correct place at the correct time doing the correct action.
- The immovable object and the unstoppable force cannot both exist. Within a relationship sometimes you have to change your approach because if you do not there will only be negative results.
- When yang is at its height we should prepare for the time when yin will come back to its own power, and vice versa.
- The universe created you but you are not controlled by it. You have free will, but heaven will reward you with a positive environment if you live in tune with the Way.
- Heaven has set a path for you, but through proper positioning and action you can greatly increase your success within the world.
- The concept of *wuwei* ("absence of action") means that you should take no forced actions in a given situation.
- *Wuwei* does not mean doing nothing. You must work hard toward your goal. Think of it as walking purposefully along a path without trying to run ahead or turn off it, no matter what comes at you.
- To "remain in the circle" means to not try to force your situation in a particular direction, but instead focus your mind back to the centre.
- There are four types of action: action (being busy), inaction (being lazy), directed action (pursuing goals) and responsive action (living life naturally and reacting to events).
- Simplicity, going with the flow and internal focus are the three main aspects of the Way.

- The Dao does not make mistakes. You are exactly where you need to be to learn.

- Your emotions should be like a deep ocean, silent and slow, not like a raging storm.

- The three steps of the Way are: *wuwei* (attention to the situation at hand), *shu* (the skills you need to deal with situations) and *yin* (basic survival ability). We should use *wuwei* and *shu* if possible and only fall back on *yin* as a last resort.

- A standard human is only instinctual. A superior human is educated and understands proper social behaviour. A sage is beyond human society and understands the foundation of the universe and correct action in all situations.

- Heaven is waiting to reward you, so if something is wrong in your life it is because you are not doing the correct thing.

- Aim to become the dragon, emblem of perfect wisdom.

BECOMING THE DRAGON

In yinyang, life is about stripping away complications. To become the dragon it is enough to follow the path laid out in this book. You can do this either in its own right or by gaining a deeper understanding of a related subject such as *feng shui*, martial arts or Traditional Chinese Medicine. No matter which way you travel, you are sure to reach the mouth of the dragon's lair – if you tread the path correctly.

I hope that you will have been encouraged to start your journey into a world that was previously unknown to you or, if you were already acquainted with these ancient Asian ideas, that you will be able to use this book to help you explain these ways to others. No matter what your approach to these ancient teachings, stay true to the path and become the dragon.

ANY MISTAKES ARE MINE

When dealing with ancient systems like yinyang, there are always issues with variations and historical mistakes of interpretation, translation or transliteration. I have attempted to "iron out" those mistakes and draw attention to alternative versions. However, if I have introduced into this book any mistakes that are not historical variations or debates between systems, then I apologize in full.

BIBLIOGRAPHY

Allinson, R. E. (editor), *Understanding the Chinese Mind: The Philosophical Roots.* Oxford University Press, Hong Kong, 1989.

Augier, S., *Urban Violence: Mian Xiang (Face Reading) for Self Defence.* Line of Intent Books, Cambridge, 2017.

Chan, W., *A Sourcebook in Chinese Philosophy.* Princeton University Press, Princeton, NJ, 1963.

Chen, Y., "Legitimation Discourse and the Theory of the Five Elements in Imperial China", *Journal of Song-Yuan Studies*, Volume 44. Society for Song, Yuan and Conquest Dynasty Studies, 2014.

Cummins, A., *The Ultimate Art of War: A Step-by-Step Illustrated Guide to Sun Tzu's Teachings.* Watkins, London, 2019.

Cummins, A. & M. Koizumi, *The Lost Samurai School: Secrets of Mubyoshi Ryu.* Blue Snake Books, Berkeley, CA, 2016.

Cummins, A. & Y. Minami, *The Book of Ninja: The First Complete Translation of the Bansenshukai.* Watkins, London, 2013.

Cummins, A. & Y. Minami, *The Book of Samurai: Fundamental Teachings* (*Book of Samurai* series, book 1). Watkins, London, 2015.

Cummins, A. & Y. Minami, *Iga and Koka Ninja Skills: The Secret Shinobi Scrolls of Chikamatsu Shigenori.* History Press, Cheltenham, Gloucs, 2013.

Cummins, A. & Y. Minami, *Samurai Arms, Armour & the Tactics of Warfare* (*Book of Samurai* series, book 2). Watkins, London, 2018.

Cummins, A. & Y. Minami, *The Secret Traditions of the Shinobi: Hattori Hanzo's Shinobi Hiden and Other Ninja Scrolls.* Blue Snake Books, Berkeley, CA, 2012.

Cummins, A. & Y. Minami, *True Path of the Ninja: The Definitive Translation of the Shoninki.* Tuttle, North Clarendon, VT, 2011.

Gentz, J. & D. Meyer (editors), *Literary Forms of Argument in Early China.* Brill, Leiden, Netherlands, 2015.

Herman, J., *Taoism for Dummies.* John Wiley & Sons, New York, 2013.

Huang, A., *The Complete I Ching: The Definitive Translation.* Inner Traditions, Rochester, VT, 1998.

Jarmey, C., *Shiatsu: Foundation Course.* Godsfield Press, Basingstoke, Hants, 1999.

Kaibara, Ekiken (author), Scott-Wilson, W. (translator), *Yojokun: Life Lessons from a Samurai.* Kodansha International, New York, 2008.

Lai, K., *An Introduction to Chinese Philosophy.* Cambridge University Press, Cambridge, 2008.
Lai, K., *Leaning from Chinese Philosophies: Ethics of Interdependent and Contextualised Self.* Ashgate, Farnham, Surrey, 2006.
Lao Tzu (author), R. A. Dale (translator), *Tao Te Ching: A New Translation and Commentary.* Watkins, London, 2002.
Leaman, O., *Encyclopedia of Asian Philosophy.* Routledge, London, 2001.
Leibniz, G. W. (author), D. J. Cook & H. Rosemont, Jr. (translators and editors), *Writings on China.* Open Court Books, Chicago and LaSalle, IL, 1994.
Li, Z. (author), M. Bell Samei (translator), *The Chinese Aesthetic Tradition.* University of Hawaii Press, Honolulu, HI, 2010.
Liu, J., *An Introduction to Chinese Philosophy: From Ancient Philosophy to Chinese Buddhism.* Blackwell Books, Oxford, 2006.
Palmer, M., *Lines of Destiny: How to Read Faces and Hands the Chinese Way.* Shambhala, Boston, MA, 1986.
Ritsema, R. & S. H. Sabbadini, *The Original I Ching Oracle or the Book of Changes.* Watkins, London, 2005.
Rochat de la Vallée, E., *The Five Elements in Chinese Classical Texts.* Monkey Press, UK, 2009.
Rochat de la Vallée, E., *Yin Yang in Classical Texts.* Monkey Press, UK, 2006.
Schwartz, B. I., *The World of Thought in Ancient China.* Belknap Press, Cambridge, MA, 1985.
Stepaniants, M., *Introduction to Eastern Thought.* AltaMira Press, Walnut Creek, CA, 2002.
Struthers, J., *The Palmistry Bible: The Definitive Guide to Hand Reading.* Godsfield Press, Basingstoke, Hants, 2005.
Tai, S., *Principles of Feng Shui: An Illustrated Guide to Chinese Geomancy.* Asiapac Books, Singapore, 1998.
Trapp, J., *Chinese Astrology: Understanding Your Horoscope.* Amber Books, London, 2015.
Wang, R. R., *Yinyang: The Way of Heaven and Earth in Chinese Thought and Culture.* Cambridge University Press, Cambridge, 2012.
Wilhelm, R., *The Secret of the Golden Flower: A Chinese Book of Life.* Harcourt, Brace & Co., New York, 1931.
Yutang, L., *The Importance of Living.* William Heinemann Ltd, London, 1938.
Zhu B. & H. Wang (editors), *Basic Theories of Traditional Chinese Medicine.* People's Military Medical Press, Beijing, 2008.

INDEX

NOTE: page numbers in **bold** refer to diagrams, page numbers in *italics* refer to information contained in tables.

D

E

F

G

H

I

J

K

L

M

N

O

P

X

Y

Z

ABOUT THE AUTHOR

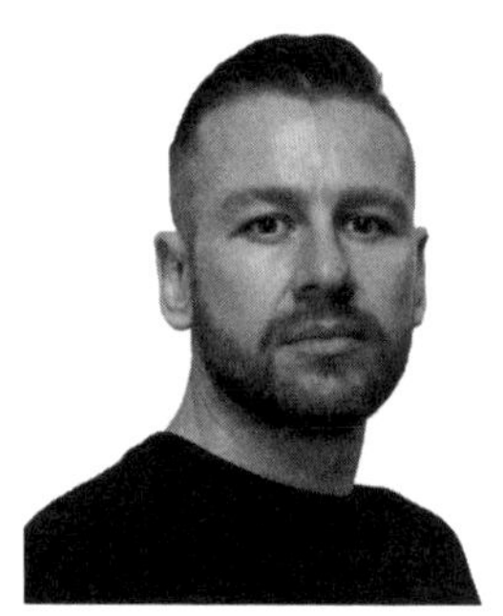

Antony Cummins is the Official Tourism Ambassador for Wakayama, Japan (和歌山市観光発信人) and an author on historical Asian military culture, specifically Japanese. His intention is to present a historically accurate picture of both samurai and *shinobi* (ninja) to the western world and lay down the foundations for a better understanding of their teachings and ways. He has published an array of books on Japanese warfare, including translations of historical ninja manuals with his translation partners. Antony and his work can be followed on YouTube under "Antony Cummins" and "Natori Ryu", as well as on Instagram under @natoriryu. For more information see his website: www.natori.co.uk

ABOUT THE ILLUSTRATOR

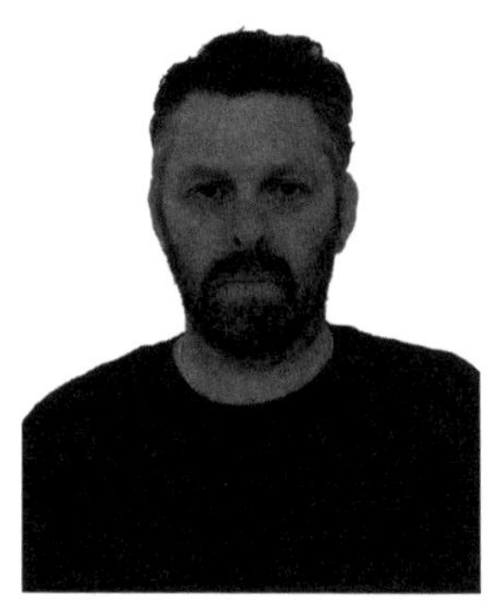

Jayson Kane is a Manchester-based graphic designer and illustrator, otherwise known as Kane Kong Illustrates (@kanekongillustrates on Instagram). He studied Art, Design and Print Making specializing in Visual Communication. Having worked with Antony Cummins for many years, his portfolio includes: *True Path of the Ninja* (cover concept design), *The Secret Traditions of the Shinobi* (front cover design), *Iga and Koka Ninja Skills* (internal illustrations), *The Illustrated Guide to Viking Martial Arts* (internal illustrations), *Ninja Skills* (internal illustrations), *Old Japan* (internal illustrations), *Modern Ninja Warfare* (internal illustrations), *The Old Stones* (internal diagrams), *The Ultimate Art of War* (internal illustrations) and *How to Be a Modern Samurai* (internal illustrations).

JOIN A SAMURAI SCHOOL OF WAR

Natori-Ryu is a samurai school of war which follows the teachings of Natori Sanjuro Masazumi – also known as Issui-sensei. The ancient scrolls and ways of war have been translated into English in the *Book of Samurai* series and the school is always open to new members who wish to follow the ancient path of the samurai. Visit www.natori.co.uk to read all about Natori-Ryu and find out how you can become a student.

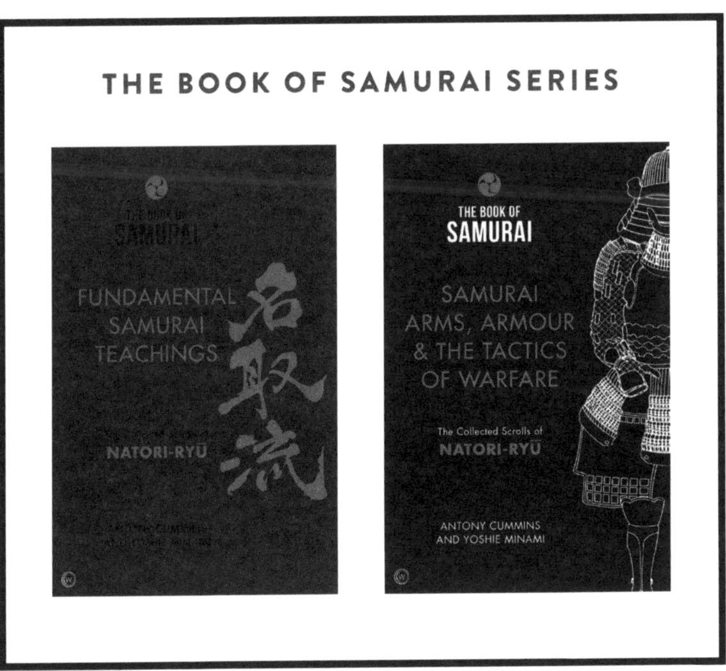